The Living Wetsuit

Demystifying anatomy for everyday use

Sue Adstrum PhD

First published 2021 by Integrative Anatomy Solutions

Produced by Indie Experts P/L, Australasia
indieexperts.com.au

Cover design and internal illustrations by Daniela Catucci @ Catucci Design
Edited by Anne-Marie Tripp
Internal design by Indie Experts
Typeset in 11.75/16 pt Kepler Std by Post Pre-press Group, Brisbane

The author would like to thank the copyright holder for their permission to reprint an excerpt from the following material: *MORTAL LESSONS: NOTES ON THE ART OF SURGERY* by Richard Selzer. Copyright © 1974, 1975, 1976, 1987 by Richard Selzer. Reprinted by permission of Georges Borchardt, Inc., on behalf of the author.

ISBN 978-0-473-70831-3 (paperback)
ISBN 978-0-473-70832-0 (epub)

Disclaimer: The information contained in this book is for educational purposes only, and is not intended to diagnose, treat, cure, or prevent any condition or disease. This book does not substitute professional medical advice. Please consult with your physician or healthcare provider for individually tailored medical advice, diagnoses, or treatment. The author, publishers, and their respective employees and agents are not responsible or liable for any injuries or damage occasioned to any person as a result of reading or following the information contained in this book. The use of this book implies your acceptance of this disclaimer.

Contents

In loving memory of
Keith Walter Hubbard (1926–1967)
who taught me about the importance of
questioning the things we presume to be true.

Preface

Anatomical dissection typically entails separating the mishmash of parts inside a chemically preserved dead body, so that they can be individually revealed and examined. One of the main tasks in dissection involves cleaning away the unnaturally opaque, dehydrated fascial tissue that connects and conceals everything else. It is next to impossible to clearly see anything (e.g., nerves, muscles) until this whitish substance has been removed and discarded. This type of cleaning is a time-consuming process that requires considerable care and patience. As medical student Christine Montross (2007, p. 247) explains, the fascia:

> clears away differently in different places. Its consistency – and hence its tenacity – varies. Under the skin it is webby and soft, and you can push through it with your flattened hand or a finger inserted between muscles. In areas of fat, it is also soft, but thick; using rat-tooth forceps, you can "pick" it away if it is in globules. If it is less dense, a whole area will fade into one clingy strand, much as a spiderweb does when you grab it with a broom. Clearing this kind of fascia makes a sound like peeling a slightly green banana. It is quiet, and one of the parts of anatomy I find most satisfying. Progress is clear, and you don't have to battle; each movement is an act of revealing – the thick belly of a gray-brown muscle, the shiny white of tendon, the gloss of smooth muscle in an organ… Other areas of fascia are tedious. The thick aponeurosis of the palm is replicated on the sole of the foot and is very slow going in both spots.

Setting the scene

Outside, the university area of Dunedin hummed with the start of the 1972 academic year. The clock at the front of the room silently informed us, the year's new physiotherapy class, that it was now just past 2 pm. A slim, white coat clad young doctor introduced himself as our first-year anatomy instructor. He would be teaching us about the body's physical structure. Anatomy is important, he said, because anatomy acts as the platform of facts that would support *everything else* we were going to learn about physiotherapy and medicine.

Until then I didn't know what anatomy was (remember, one couldn't ask Google in those days), only that it must be a really big subject, as it took up lots of space in our course timetable. Studying anatomy, he told us, was going to occupy a huge amount of our time and energy for the next three years. Failing any of our frequent anatomy exams was not an option if we wished to continue our training. If we couldn't master anatomy, we would be expelled.

Next, he asked for someone, a volunteer, to tell him what the body is. We were going to be studying them, so what are they? The room's silence instantly deepened a couple more notches. Not daring to look around to see what anyone else was doing, I held my breath, and studiously stared down at my notepad. In truth, I felt stupid, and uncomfortable. His question sounded so easy, yet, to my surprise, I was unable to answer it. So, right then and there (still avoiding his gaze), I promised myself that I'd study this subject as hard as I possibly could. I wanted to make sure I would pass all of those now-dreaded anatomy exams – which may well have been the point of his asking that question.

Winning the student anatomy prize three years later was a happy graduation day surprise. Yet there were some even better rewards in store. Somewhere along the way, those days and nights of hard work had dissolved my fear of this subject and ignited my brand-new passion for it. Anatomy plays some enormously helpful roles in the world, and I wanted in on them. Even though I was just a beginner, I now knew the basic rules of the game ... and willingly signed on as a player. And, best of all, the overcoming-the-fear side of things had revealed the value of being kind to one's students when, many years later, it was my turn to teach others – some of whom were as, if not more, frightened than I had been that 1972 afternoon. Sharing their joy as they came to grips with their studies, and then nailed their exams, was priceless. And now, being able to help people from many different walks of life discover that anatomy is *really* interesting, *really* important ... and that it is possible for them all to learn about these things in an easy and fun manner.

Bodies and anatomy

"Anatomy. The science of bodily structure. Structure as discovered by dissection. The body of facts and deductions as to the structure of organised beings, animal or vegetable, ascertained by dissection. The doctrine or science of structure. From the French 'anatomie'. From the Latin 'anatomia'. From the Greek 'anatomia' [ἀνατομία]. 'Ana' [ἀνά], up. 'Toma' [τομ-], cut." *(Roberts, 2021)*

So, how would you fare if someone asked *you* the same question? How easily could you explain what your body is to a stranger wearing a white coat? Don't worry, you are definitely not alone if you think you might have some difficulty doing this.

Strange as it might seem, many health professionals, scientists, university scholars, educators, and health system administrators would also have difficulty with this task. Large parts of their work involve directly and indirectly caring for, studying, writing and or teaching about people's bodies – which means that they all need to know something about the body's structural makeup. They know what they were once taught, as were their teachers before them. The validity of their ideas about this subject is generally taken for granted, but it has rarely, if ever, been formally examined (Birke, 1999). This almost universal lack of critical attention to so important a subject ought to be a matter of serious concern – especially when there are some significant shortcomings in what we have traditionally been taught.

Health professionals – acupuncturists, bodywork and movement therapists, chiropractors, dentists, dieticians, doctors, massage therapists, midwives, naturopaths, nurses, occupational therapists, optometrists, osteopaths, paramedics, podiatrists, pharmacists, physiotherapists, and surgeons, to name but a few of many – clearly need to learn about anatomy in great (and, for some, very great) detail. Yet, if you were to ask them to define what the body means to them, they could well look at you sideways, as if you'd asked them a trick question (Nicholls, 2018). These people work with bodies so much, and so often, that the human body has become something quite ordinary. So ordinary that their particular knowledge of it is frequently hidden from view.

Before going any further, please realise it's easy to feel confused by the word *anatomy*. A lot of this can be blamed on it being a multiuse word that variably refers to several quite different things (see Table 0.1), all of which have something to do with describing the body's structure with a certain sort of meaning in mind. The problem is that people tend to assume that everyone else instinctively knows which meaning they are referring to when they use this word. As this assumption is not always correct, the different meanings have sometimes gotten a bit mixed up and muddled.

The scientific art of describing the body's structural makeup.

A formally taught curriculum subject that teaches students about the body's anatomical structure.

An internationally agreed-upon set of knowledge (i.e., concepts and representations) that bioscientifically describes the body's physical structure.

One of many socio-culturally agreed-upon sets of knowledge (i.e., concepts and representations) that systematically describe the body's structural make-up (plural, *anatomies*).

An occupational profession that scientifically describes the body's anatomical structure.

Book purpose and book structure

Our bodies are a big and important part of who we are. They are always with us while we're alive. They are involved in and affect everything we can and cannot do. Everyone – not just university educated 'experts' and health professionals – can benefit from learning more about their body's structure, because it relates to the ways we care for it and, when needs be, help it to heal. If we understand the basics, we are well positioned to apply this knowledge to improving our own – as well as our patients', employees', and families' – everyday health and wellbeing. It is therefore really helpful that our knowledge of our body is as accurate and up to date as possible. This book shows that obtaining this knowledge need not be a difficult task – it actually can be quite easy and enjoyable.

In today's Western medical system, the body is widely construed as a machine-like assemblage of supposedly separate biological body parts – such as muscles and bones, visceral organs, and fluid transporting vessels (Nicholls, 2018). From this way of looking at things, the fascia (the body's soft connective tissue) that links everything together and makes the body whole – as Nature intended it to be – is generally overlooked and forgotten about. This conventional way of thinking – i.e., where body parts are regarded as body-machine components – has supported the development and widespread use of surgery, pharmaceutical medicines, and musculoskeletal body treatments. Many of us, myself included, have periodically benefited from this way of conceptualising the body – even though, as many anatomists as well as many scientists and health professionals now know, it is not entirely accurate or complete.

In reality, our bodies are not machines that have been built from a collection of separate parts. They are far more wonderful and interesting than that. Our bodies are naturally whole and alive. Everything inside them is interconnected and important, including the fascia that enables all of their so-called 'parts' to dynamically work together in a cohesive manner. Acknowledging the body's innate wholeness and aliveness makes it possible for us to adjust and hopefully improve the ways we heal and look after it, for instance, through our additional use of fascia-relating bodywork and movement therapies. This can be incredibly useful, especially if we are grappling with some persistent and seemingly difficult to resolve health and pain problems.

This book is designed for a well-educated general or lay audience – although I hope it may also be useful to a diverse range of health professionals, health educators, health researchers, and health system managers. It uses easy to understand language to address three main subjects – anatomy, fascia, and the Living Wetsuit – all three of which are conceptually connected to our bodies, as well as to each other. This book deliberately approaches these subjects from a big-picture (transdisciplinary) perspective[1] that helps us to see that our understanding of these things is contextualised by the time and place the knowledge was constructed. As you will soon see, there are many ways of thinking about each of them, and their linkages to each other.

The first section of this book broadly deals with the subject of anatomy – our knowledge of the body's structure. Anatomy

1 My university studies in anatomy, anthropology, medical history, and public health enabled me to develop an integrative anatomical way of looking at the body that combines the systems of thought usually associated with these science and humanities disciplines. This unconventionally broad, multiple-discipline-spanning viewpoint makes it possible to talk about bodies and fascia in a biologically- *and* historically- *and* socially-contextualised manner. This is particularly helpful when explaining complex phenomena, and when developing innovative solutions for some of society's difficult to solve health problems.

matters because, as Chapter 1 explains, it underpins our understanding of how the body works and might best be cared for. Differing sets of anatomical knowledge justify different types of health care. History shows us that different sets of anatomical knowledge (anatomies, Chapter 2) are shaped by different methods of observation, therapeutic experience, textual tradition, religious and philosophical ideas, and the ways people generally live in the world at a particular time in history. This means there are many ways human bodies can be understood and explained, all of which are liable to change and evolve with the passage of time. Each one potentially adds to our cumulative understanding of what the body is, though none of them, on their own, can do this fully. Chapter 3 shows how, in the Western medical tradition, the development of anatomical knowledge has relied heavily on the scientific examination of dissected cadavers (anatomised corpses). This research approach has been extremely valuable, as it has helped us learn a considerable amount about the position and structure of the body's seemingly separate interior parts. Recent advances in research technology are now making it possible for anatomists to also 'observe' the insides of bodies that are alive and intact, without cutting them into pieces. These new technology-enhanced views are valuably expanding our knowledge of the body's structural makeup and providing some valuable new insights about the ways our bodies work and move.

The middle section of this book deals with the subject of fascia – fascia (Chapter 4) and fascial anatomy (Chapter 5). Twentieth century anatomists generally perceived fascia as a relatively unimportant body part. As a result, it was not comprehensively described in the anatomical research literature, and was routinely omitted from most downstream scientific, professional, scholarly, and public understandings of bodily structure. This oversight, as understandable as it is, has (inevitably) limited the ways we have been able to think about caring for and remedially treating a (hypothetically fascia-less) body form. This situation has changed considerably during the past decades – ever since fascia became the focus of an emerging field of interdisciplinary research enquiry. Adding fascia back into the picture has valuably expanded our understanding of the body as well as the things we might do to look after and heal it.

The third and biggest section of this book (Chapter 6) starts out by introducing the concept of the Living Wetsuit (LWS), the body's soft and life-energy-infused, skeleton-hugging garment. Chapter 7 describes the biological fabric that forms into the LWS. We wear our LWSs for all of our lives. They get a lot of use, hence can sometimes become a bit damaged or unwell. Chapter 8 looks at some of the things that can adversely affect the LWS, and what consequently happens to it. On a happier note, Chapter 9 explains some of the things that we can do to look after and to help heal the LWS. The final chapter, Chapter 10, situates the LWS in our 21st century world environment. The way the world thinks about the body and its fascia has evolved over millennia, and is continuing to evolve. Our knowledge of anatomy, fascia and the LWS is extremely important, and advances in technology have helped change it substantially during the past few decades. This matters because our understanding of these things powerfully influences the ways we are (individually and collectively) now able to think about, and be actively involved in, our bodies' health and health care – even if we are not aware that this is happening. The LWS analogy helps demystify anatomy. It explains our body's structure in a scientifically accurate, yet simple and easy to understand manner. It also gives us all – both lay people and health experts – a tool we can use to help improve our health, and that of the people we care for.

Finally, at the end of all of this, there is a glossary that defines some of the specialised terms that have been used in this book and may seem a bit strange to some readers.

Anatomy Matters

01

An important tipping point

Andries van Wesel was born in Brussels in the winter of 1514. He was born during the Renaissance, a time in history when the people of Europe were experiencing a great deal of change in their lives. This was a time when many of the usual, old-style ways of thinking about and doing things were challenged and updated. Vast changes were seen in Europe's art, for instance, as well as its music, mathematics, medicine, and religion. For young Andries, this was an exciting time to be born into.

Eighteen-year-old Andries began his university studies in Paris, and soon developed a passion for anatomy. Anatomy was then viewed as part of a well-rounded academic education, so it was studied by many different types of students – not just those preparing for a medical career. Andries took an especially keen interest in the classes taught by Jacques Dubois (Sylvius).[2] Sylvius was an orthodox anatomist, so his teaching was in keeping with the ways the body had been earlier explained by Galen of Pergamon. Galen (c. 130–c. 210 AD) was an eminent Greek-born Roman physician, surgeon and philosopher whose many medical successes were supported by his ground-breaking anatomy research. At that time, Roman law had prohibited the

A tipping point is the moment at which a series of small happenings sets off a large and important change in the world.

2 During the European Renaissance (14th–17th century), scholars, who came from many different countries, generally discussed each other's ideas in Latin – a language they could all understand. As a result, many prominent scholars, including anatomists, were internationally known by Latinised versions of their names. Jacques Dubois (1478–1555), a French anatomist, for example, was referred to as *Jacobus Sylvius*, or *Sylvius*; and Thomas Bartholin (1616–1680), an anatomist from Denmark, became known as *Thomas Bartholinus,* or *Bartholinus*.

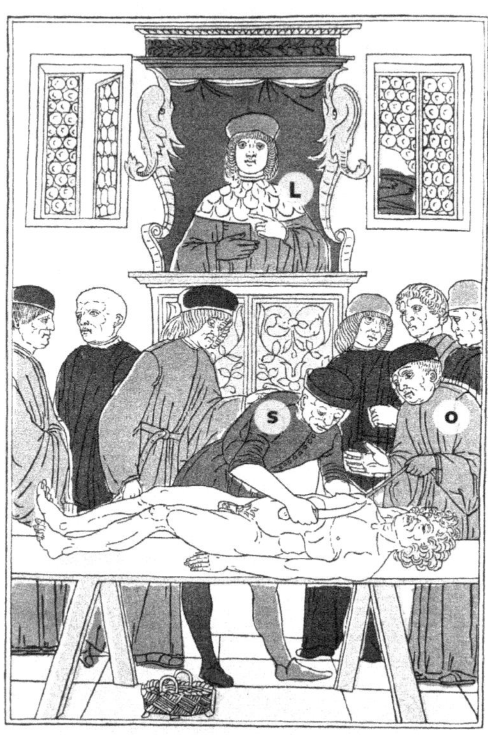

Figure 1.1
Anatomical dissection
in the 15th century

In 1238, Frederick II, the Holy Roman Emperor, issued an edict requiring surgeons to study anatomy, and ordered the first public dissection of a judicially executed criminal's corpse to help them do so. Over time, the witnessing of such a dissection was increasingly used to reinforce Galen's classical anatomy doctrine. For several hundred years, the dissections were performed by a three-member team (as shown in this 15th century woodcut): (1) the professor of anatomy (Lector, **L**) sat in a prominent position away from the corpse, where he could easily be heard as he read from the textbook in front of him; (2) the Sector (**S**), usually a surgeon, dissected the body; and (3) the demonstrator (Ostensor, **O**) used a rod to point to the parts of the body the Lector was describing.

dissection of human cadavers (dead people's bodies), so Galen dissected the bodies of live animals – including dogs, monkeys, and pigs (Standring, 2016a). Like many of his colleagues, he also studied what he could see through the gaps of his patients' wounds and the surgical incisions he made in their flesh. Galen passed on his many new ideas and discoveries through his teaching, and a large amount of scholarly writing. His texts were so highly regarded and useful that they were widely circulated and copied many times over. Those that survived Western Europe's cultural descent into the Dark Ages (many didn't) were translated into Arabic, and from Arabic into medieval Latin, powerfully influencing the ways people (including Sylvius) thought about anatomy for most of the next 1,500 years.

As his studies progressed, Andries became increasingly frustrated with Sylvius's style of teaching. Simply put, Sylvius – along with most of his predecessors, peers, and the Catholic Church – firmly believed that Galen had been inspired by God, which basically meant that Galen's knowledge of anatomy was holy, could not be faulted, and would never require any improvement. Sylvius consequently taught anatomy in the traditional manner – by restating and interpreting Galen's age-old ideas. Following Galen's lead, he only used the carcasses of animals – never human cadavers – in his anatomy demonstrations (see Figure 1.1). Any troublesome discrepancies between the book and the corpse in front of him were blamed on the corpse. Galen was, at least as far as Sylvius was concerned, an infallible authority!

Andries and his friends' extracurricular trips to look at the piles of human bones stored in a nearby cemetery's ossuary showed that the structure of some bones – such as the mandible (or jawbone) and sacrum – regularly differed from the way Galen had described them many centuries earlier. Andries worried that Sylvius's loyalty to Galen's ideas prevented him from examining and explaining these seeming 'discrepancies' in bone structure. Was it possible that Galen's descriptions of human anatomy might not have been as perfect as most people, especially Sylvius, seemed to think they were?

War intervened and Andries returned home to Belgium, where he completed his bachelor's degree. He then obtained his doctorate in medicine at Italy's University of Padua. His moving there had a lot to do with Italy's more progressive attitude to anatomical dissection. Living in Italy gave him access to a plentiful supply of human cadavers that he could lawfully dissect, after their original owners had met their life's end at the gallows.

Andreas Vesalius, or Vesalius, as he was now internationally known, chose to perform his public anatomy dissections all by himself (see Figure 1.2). He spoke off the cuff rather than reading from a book, he got his hands dirty, and personally pointed to the body parts he was describing. Vesalius's research reinforced many of Galen's earlier findings, and also enabled him to correct some of Galen's unintentional descriptive errors. His unconventional approach to anatomy attracted its critics, vociferously including Sylvius, as well as a rapidly growing number of supporters. Vesalius's first two books[3] were published in 1543, shortly before his 30th birthday. As far as is known, these were the world's first technically accurate anatomy textbooks. They famously included a specially commissioned (and soon to be much plagiarised) set of highly detailed and accurate anatomical drawings. Both books, and in particular their artwork, were

[3] *De Humani Corporis Fabrica Libri Septum* ('On the Fabric of the Human Body in Seven Books'); and *De Humani Corporis Fabrica Librorum Epitome*, an illustrated compendium volume commonly known as the *Epitome*.

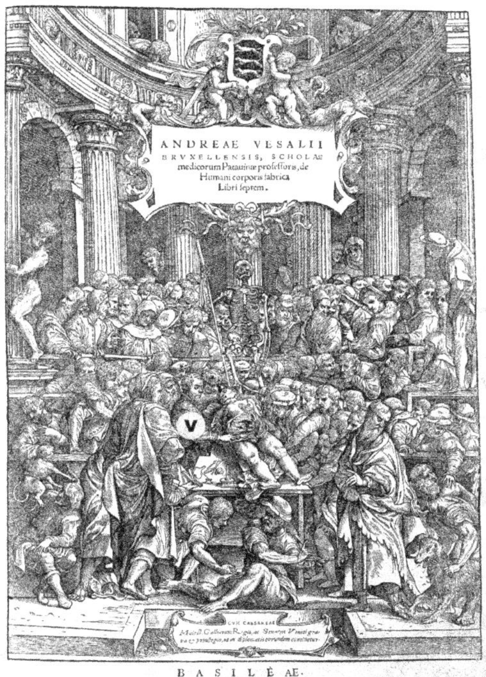

Figure 1.2
Vesalius-style anatomy
dissection

The title page of Vesalius's *De Humani Corporis Fabrica* (published in Switzerland in 1543) portrays its author (Vesalius, **V**) conducting a public anatomy dissection, in which he personally did all of the dissecting, pointing things out, and teaching.

instantly and enormously successful, and played an influential role in the promotion of a new, scientific dissection-based, system of human anatomical knowledge.

Why anatomy matters

Vesalius didn't do all of this because he wanted to show off how clever he was. He didn't set out to show up Galen's mistakes. He did it because he understood that the ways we understand and think about our bodies' structure is vitally important to *us all*. He knew, as did many of his esteemed predecessors, that people's knowledge of anatomy conceptually supports their practices of health care and healing.

Anatomy matters because a group of people's understanding of the body's structure affects the ways they *are able to* think about health care and medicine. Anatomy serves as the theoretical foundation of medicine. It is a conceptual point of departure for all types of medical and surgical care, as well as the in-between understandings of physiology and pathology that support them (see Figure 1.3).

It is therefore important to ensure that our anatomical knowledge is as accurate and up to date as possible, and not allowed to become something that we were once taught and now unthinkingly take for granted. If it happened to Vesalius and Sylvius, it is possible there may have been some outdated ideas in what *our* teachers conveyed to us.[4]

4 Anatomical knowledge is continually evolving, as are educational curricula. Still, there can be a lag between the time of a research discovery and its translation into a curriculum (and textbook) change.

Anatomy is important because our knowledge of the body's structure:

1. Enables us to explain how the body normally works (physiology)
2. Helps us understand how the body is affected by injury and disease (pathology)
3. Powerfully shapes the ways we are able to think about our bodies' health and health care.

Vesalius also, very importantly, found out that *anatomical knowledge is constructed by people*, not by the God who (as everyone then believed) created their bodies. This meant that people's knowledge of anatomy is not necessarily going to be perfect and consistent. It is also likely to develop and change as new information comes to hand.

What Vesalius did mattered a lot. He did far more than developing some new anatomy facts, and showing anatomy ought to be taught from human bodies as well as from books. His unplanned discovery that people's knowledge of anatomy can change and be improved on over time was then revolutionary. His new findings and ideas were welcomed by many of his peers, yet they also met with a fair bit of resistance from others, because they challenged what had long been the usual way of thinking about the body and anatomy. So much so, that it took well over a century before his way of thinking was generally accepted as correct. Even though it took this long to be established, Vesalius's ground-breaking work helped *tip the balance* from the ways people had thought anatomy was for a very long time to something that was better, and more in-tune with the giant changes that were then sweeping through Renaissance society. It can be seen as *a tipping point* that set off some large and important changes in the worlds of anatomy and medicine that have continued to develop through to our present day.

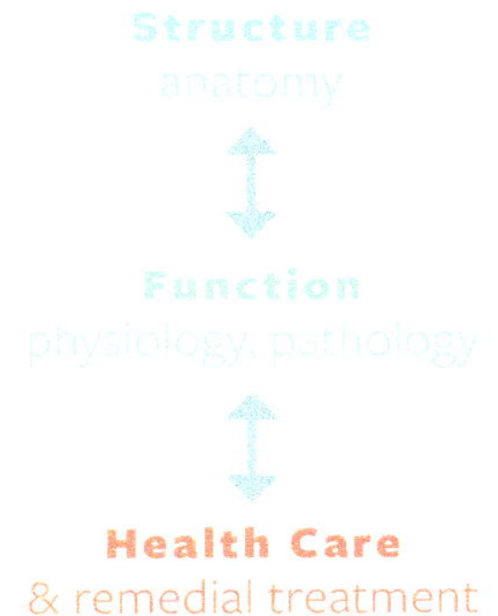

Figure 1.3
Anatomy matters

Understanding the body's anatomical structure makes it possible to explain how the body works, what happens when it is hurt or unwell, and what can be done to protect and improve its health.

Anatomy and influenza

The evolving connection between anatomy and medicine can be seen, for example, in the differing ways that a widespread and lethal outbreak of influenza was medically dealt with shortly before, and then again nearly 500 years after, Vesalius's 16th century lifetime. The different understandings of anatomy in both of these periods underpin two quite different types (systems) of health care.

The world's first documented influenza pandemic suddenly appeared and spread all through Europe during the summer of 1510. This febrile coughing disease was soon known by quite a few names, including *das Gruppe* (German for 'the group', because most people got it), and *Coccoluche* or *Coccolucio* (from the Latin *culcullus* meaning 'hood', as sufferers often tried to ease their headache by covering their head with a hood). It was varyingly defined as: a precipitous illness with coughing and a high fever (by a lawyer/politician); a respiratory catarrh with cardiac and pulmonary constriction and coughing (by a king's physician); and a rheumatic affliction of the head with constriction of the head and lungs (by an anatomist/surgeon) (Morens et al., 2010). A Dr. Short later reported (in Thompson, 1852, pp. 3–4, emphasis in original) that the pandemic "attacked at once, and raged all over *Europe*, not missing a family, and scarce a person." In his words, the illness typically began with a "grievous pain in the head, heaviness, difficulty of breathing, hoarseness, loss of strength and appetite, restlessness, watchings [inability to sleep], from a terrible taring cough." These symptoms were soon followed by

> a chilness [sic], and so a violent cough, that many were in danger of suffocation. The first few days it was without spitting; but about the seventh or eighth day, much viscid phlegm was spit up. Others (though fewer,) spit only water and froth. When they began to spit, cough and shortness of

breath were easier ... In some, it went off with a looseness [diarrhoea]; in others, by sweating.

At that time, medicine was officially practiced by a socially elite group of physicians.[5] Their treatment methods were based on an age-old belief (powerfully endorsed by Hippocrates, Aristotle, Galen, and Ibn Sina, for example) that related health to the balanced working of a person's soul, mind, and physical body. From this perspective, the body's structure and functioning were described in relation to four different types of body sap or juice, known as humoral fluids (blood, phlegm, black bile, and yellow bile). Pain and poor health were blamed on an unbalanced relationship between these four humours. Medical care was accordingly aimed at restoring a more favourable humoral balance – through, for example, bloodletting, purging, geographic relocation, and dietary modification.

The physicians practicing this style of medicine needed to have a relatively sound knowledge of the structure, location, and workings of the parts of the body that were then known to materially control the body's humoral balance and health. This meant that they needed to know something about the organs (e.g., liver, spleen), fluid-secreting membranes (e.g., peritoneum, pleura), and fluid-carrying vessels (e.g., arteries, veins) in the body's abdominal, chest, and head cavities. Which, according to the texts that they wrote, just happened to be the parts of the body that most interested that era's anatomists.

Nobody then knew for sure what caused this deadly disease.[6] Many people, including the Pope in Rome, blamed it on God's anger. Physicians, however, generally described it in terms of things that were likely to have disturbed a person's humoral balance – such as the unseasonable weather, earthquakes, volcanic eruptions, plagues of locusts, or an outbreak of a dangerous cattle disease that preceded the pandemic's arrival (Thompson, 1852; Morens et al., 2010). Their medical treatments

5 The messier work – such as pulling out teeth, patching up war wounds, amputations and surgeries – was generally left to lower socially-ranking barbers and surgeons.

6 Viruses weren't discovered until the 20th century (Morens & Taubenberger, 2011).

were accordingly aimed at rectifying their individual patients' body fluid imbalances by, for example, inducing diarrhoea, perspiration, or blistering. Most of these remedies were reported to be fairly ineffectual, and some, especially bloodletting and purging, turned out to be more harmful than helpful (Thompson, 1852; Morens et al., 2010).

The first few months of 2020 were marked by the onset and rapid spread of the world's latest influenza pandemic – a highly contagious respiratory disease known as COVID-19. As in 1510, some people associated the onset of this fearful disease with a variety of spiritual and other environmental influences. The conventional, scientific medical view, however, ascribed the blame entirely to the unwelcome arrival of an extremely infectious virus (the severe acute respiratory syndrome coronavirus, or SARS-CoV-2 for short).

Most of the world's mainstream medical, scientific, economic, political, and media reports about this disease were conceptually based on a contemporary anatomical understanding of the structure and functioning of the body's organ systems, and the parts (organs, tissues, cells, and molecules) they are made of. At first, the disease was mainly portrayed as a battle between the body's respiratory (*the victim*) and immune (*the hero*) systems, and the SARS-CoV-2 virus (*the vicious villain*). Although it was soon realised that this battle could also involve the brain, heart, blood vessels, kidneys, or gut; and the immune system could overreact in its attempts to rid the body of the virus infection and unfortunately cause some other new, and at times long-lasting, health problems ('long COVID').

The disease was medically portrayed as a biological problem that could be rationally solved with modern-day medical technology (i.e., a complex raft of medicines, equipment, and procedures) and community health measures (e.g., travel restrictions, social distancing). Medical treatment was primarily focused on four fronts, which were suitably dealt with by a host of biomedical specialty professions – including, but not limited to, epidemiology, immunology, medical imaging, pathology, respiratory medicine, public health medicine, and virology. Their collective effort was aimed at:

- Reducing disease transmission by slowing or preventing the spread of the virus from people who were already carrying it to everyone else in their vicinity. This was achieved through a mix of infection testing, contact tracing and social distancing measures (intended to prevent the virus's spread between individuals, population groups, and geographic regions), and physical hygiene measures (e.g., use of hand sanitisers and hand washing, disinfecting communally shared surfaces), and the wearing of personal protective equipment (e.g., masks, gloves, body-covering garments) to prevent the spread of virus-infected body fluids.

- Easing the diverse physical symptoms of this rapid-onset influenza illness – such as a sore throat, bad cough, fever, sweating, aching muscles, headaches, tiredness, diarrhoea, skin rashes, shortness of breath, chest pain, difficulty breathing – with bed rest and paracetamol tablets, through to the provision of intravenous fluids, oxygen-enriched air, corticosteroid medication, postural lung drainage, and machine-driven breathing assistance devices.

- Disease treatment. An initial absence of specifically designed COVID-19-fighting medicines was associated with a race to develop some new ones (e.g., monoclonal antibodies, convalescent plasma therapy) or repurpose some already existing others, (e.g., Remdesivir, drugs used to treat malaria), that it was hoped might obstruct the disease's advance through an infected person's body.

- Eliminating people's susceptibility to catching and further transmitting the disease (e.g., by learning much more about the virus and the sickness it causes, by monitoring the impacts and outcomes of this disease, and through the development of effective vaccines and vaccination programmes).

When Vesalius helped change the way the world thinks about anatomy nearly 500 years ago, he helped progress the way people *could* think about everything else to do with the body. How it works when it is healthy. What happens when it is hurt or gets sick. What we can do to help it stay healthy. And, when needs be, how it can be helped to get better again. All of which are useful to know when dealing with the horribleness of an influenza pandemic, whenever one turns up in the world.

Anatomies

"There are many realities. There are many versions of what may appear obvious. Whatever appears as the unshakeable truth, its exact opposite may be true in another context. After all, one's reality is but perception, viewed through various prisms of context." *(Tripathi, 2010, p. 229)*

The blind men and the elephant

There once lived six scholarly old men who, in the middle of a thought-provoking discussion about elephants, suddenly realised that none of them truly knew what an elephant was – because none of them had actually ever seen one. So, even though they were all blind, they travelled to a place where an elephant lived. And, just as soon as each had found a comfortable space for himself, they began using their hands to examine the elephant's body (see Figure 2.1).

As a result, each scholar's knowledge of one and the same elephant was different, as all six of them had separately studied only one part of its body. They only found out about the part that was closest, and thus most easy for them to inspect – such as an ear, or a tusk, or the tail. Their focusing on that one part helped them develop some useful information about it, *but* (and this is the part they missed) it didn't tell them all that much

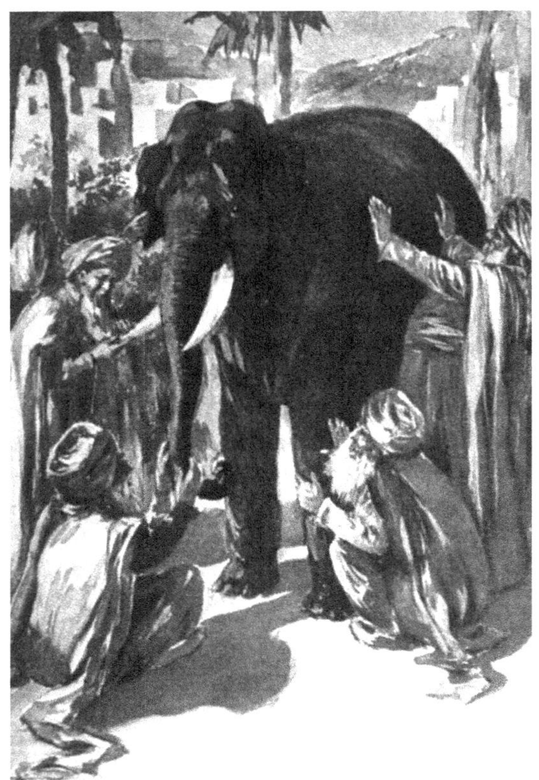

about the whole creature – which was, to be frank, far larger and far more complex than any of them realised. Each and all of them fervently believed in the truth of their discovery, yet their conclusions about the elephant's body form were (at best) quite limited, and wide of the mark, when viewed from this broader perspective.

The blind men and the elephant

It was six men of [India]
To learning much inclined,
Who went to see the Elephant
(Though all of them were blind),
That each by observation
Might satisfy his mind.

The First approached the Elephant,
And happening to fall
Against his broad and sturdy side,
At once began to bawl:
"God bless me! but the Elephant
Is very like a WALL!"

The Second, feeling of the tusk,
Cried, "Ho! what have we here,
So very round and smooth and sharp?
To me 'tis mighty clear
This wonder of an Elephant
Is very like a SPEAR!"

The Third approached the animal,
And happening to take
The squirming trunk within his hands,
Thus boldly up and spake:
"I see," quoth he, "the Elephant
Is very like a SNAKE!"

The Fourth reached out an eager hand,
And felt about the knee
"What most this wondrous beast is like
Is mighty plain," quoth he:
"'Tis clear enough the Elephant
Is very like a TREE!"

The Fifth, who chanced to touch the ear,
Said: "E'en the blindest man
Can tell what this resembles most;
Deny the fact who can,
This marvel of an Elephant
Is very like a FAN!"

The Sixth no sooner had begun
About the beast to grope,
Than seizing on the swinging tail
That fell within his scope,
"I see," quoth he, "the Elephant
Is very like a ROPE!"

And so these men of [India]
Disputed loud and long,
Each in his own opinion
Exceedingly stiff and strong,
Though each was partly in the right,
And all were in the wrong.

(Saxe, 1949, pp. 122–123)

Anatomies

As this ancient parable suggests, there's always more than one way of explaining something. That something may be an elephant. It may be a person's body. It may be how to deal with a certain type of health problem. The truth is like a revolving disco ball that reflects the light directed at it in many directions. Each of its many light-reflecting mirror glass facets has potential to tell us something – but never quite everything – about the subject at hand.

As a result, there are many different ways of conceptualising our bodies' anatomical structure – I call them *anatomies*. Each anatomy is a communally agreed-upon set of anatomical concepts and representations. Every one of them metaphorically reflects the light that has been directed at it from the society, and even a certain section of the society, it exists in. They are all shaped "in varying proportions and in different ways" by many things – including (but not only), what people in that society have been taught about anatomy, the ways the body is customarily examined and explained by their anatomists, the usual types of medical treatment, religious and philosophical ideas, political and economic circumstances, and the deep-seated "cultural imagination" (i.e., the modes of understanding, including values, laws, and symbols) shared by a particular group of people and the society they live in (Siraisi, 1995).

Our bodies are not, and are unlikely to have ever been, conceptualised in exactly the same way in every part of the world. We see this in the ways people's bodies have been anatomically portrayed and medically cared for in different countries over thousands of years – in ancient Egypt, Greece, and India; in medieval Europe and the Byzantine Empire; in Renaissance Italy and Ming Dynasty China; in precolonial Hawaii, post-colonial Africa, and in bi-cultural New Zealand. Even today, acupuncturists, brain surgeons, massage therapists, physiotherapists,

Bodies are natural. Anatomies are not. Anatomies are created and used by people.

and internal medicine physicians throughout our globalised world are quite likely to be using different, yet overlapping sets of anatomical knowledge – each of which is in keeping with the types of treatment they offer – as is evident in the following two stories.

A congenital hole in the heart, and a gateway that ought not be opened

From a Western medical perspective …

Congenital heart disease (a condition people are born with) is caused by a flaw in the heart's physical structure, such as a ventricular septal defect (VSD). A VSD is an abnormal hole in the strong muscular wall that normally separates the heart's two main blood-pumping chambers (or ventricles). If the VSD is large enough, it can disrupt the blood's normal circulation pattern through the heart and lungs, making it much harder for the heart to pump enough oxygen-rich blood throughout the body (see Figure 2.2). Over time, the extra strain can lead to the development of heart failure – a slowly worsening condition where the heart can't keep up with the body's need for oxygen-rich blood, and eventually stops working.

Diagnosis of VSD typically entails a series of medical tests, including: chest X-rays that produce images of the heart and nearby lungs and blood vessels; an electrocardiogram that records the heart's electrical activity; cardiac catheterisation, which uses a small video-camera to look at the heart's internal structure as well to check the blood pressure and blood-oxygen levels inside the heart.

The medical treatment for this condition depends upon the size, location, and severity of the hole in the heart's inner wall. It can range from doing nothing except for keeping a watchful eye on the patient's condition, using medication (e.g., to prevent

There is more than one way of explaining and treating most health problems.

bacterial infection inside the heart, to help normalise blood pressure), through to surgically closing the hole, or, in some instances, replacing the heart.

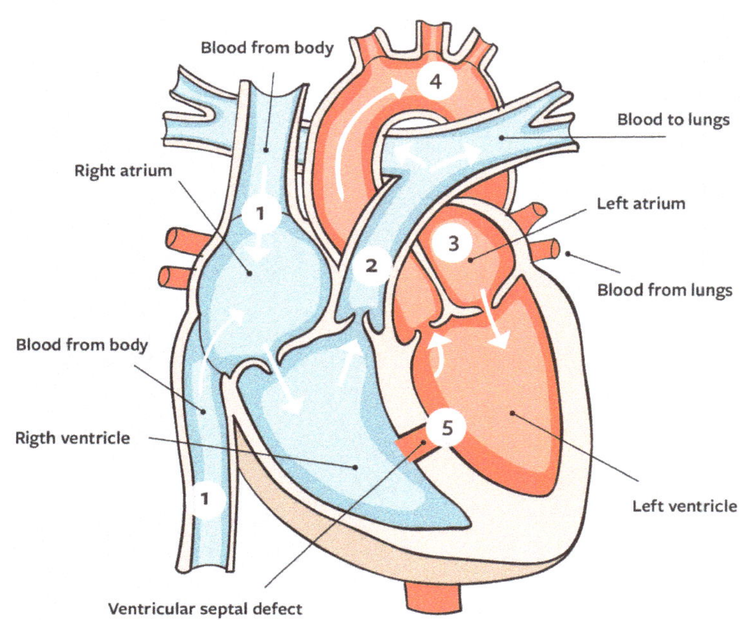

Figure 2.2
The anatomy of an interventricular septal heart defect

From a Western medical perspective, the heart is likened to a four-chambered pump that helps propel the blood circulating through the lungs and the rest of the body. The arrows show the route oxygen-poor blood (blue) normally flows as (**1**) it enters the heart's right side (on left side of diagram) from the body, and (**2**) is pumped up into the lungs to be replenished with fresh oxygen. (**3**) The now oxygen-rich blood (red) enters the left side of the heart (on the right side of the diagram), where it is pumped out through the arteries (**4**) into the rest of the body. A ventricular septal defect (**5**) is a hole in the wall between the heart's two main pumping chambers (the right and left ventricles) which abnormally allows oxygen-rich blood to pass from the left to the right side of the heart, then back through the lungs instead of out into the rest of the body.

From a Tibetan medical perspective …

In the ancient Tibetan system of anatomy and medicine, a person's body is perceived as an organised grouping of physical *and* non-physical structural elements. Some of these include the *bones, nerves, tendons, veins*, the *cord of hope*, the *religious wheel of the heart*, the *etheric body*, and the life-giving *soul* (Walsh, 1910). The body's constitution is didactically likened to an Indian fig tree that rises up through a series of trunks, stems, branches, leaves, blossoms, and fruits. Health and disease are explained in relation to a variety of intangible factors, all of which are affected by the relative condition of the body's three humours (like three entwined fig tree trunks) – wind, bile, and phlegm. In this way, the "life-keeping wind or air," for example, "resides in the upper part of the head; that which operates upward has its place in the breast; that which pervades or encompasses all resides in the heart; that which communicates or conveys an equal heat to the body has its seat in the stomach; that which cleanses downwards abides in the lowest part of the trunk" (Walsh, 1910, p. 1223).

From a Tibetan medical perspective, every person is responsible for taking care of their own health, and preventing illness from developing. This might involve a person balancing their (personal, environmental, and spiritual) relationships, modifying their diet and lifestyle, and gaining a deeper understanding of their own personality (Benor, 2004). Now and then, they may consult a medical practitioner to improve their understanding of their present state of health, and to find out what else could possibly be done do to improve it.

Tibetan medical practitioners employ a variety of sense-based techniques to evaluate their patient's physical and psychological condition – e.g., assessing a range of body pulses that can be palpated at the wrist. They may prescribe some remedies, including nutritional and lifestyle changes, herbal medicines, breathing with visualisation exercises, massage, and cupping (Walsh, 1910; Benor, 2004). Their main goal, however, is to awaken their patient's innate self-healing abilities, which may necessitate the medical practitioner entering a highly refined and compassionate level of consciousness. Spiritually advanced physician-priests or lamas may also personally intervene and contribute to the healing process, but only after the physical and emotional aspects of the problem have been attended to (Benor, 2004). This traditional Tibetan approach to diagnosis and healing is illustrated in the following account, which was written by the late Richard Selzer, an American surgeon and author (1976, pp. 33–36):

> On the bulletin board in the front hall of the hospital where
> I work, there appeared an announcement. "Yeshi Dhonden,"
> it read, "will make rounds at six o'clock in the morning of

June 10th." The particulars were given, followed by a notation: "Yeshi Dhonden is personal physician to the Dalai Lama."

I am not so leathery a skeptic that I would knowingly ignore an emissary from the gods. Not only might such sang-froid be inimical to one's earthly well-being, it could take care of eternity as well. Thus, on the morning of June 10th, I join the clutch of whitecoats waiting in the small conference room adjacent to the ward selected for the round. The air was heavy with ill-concealed dubiety and suspicion of bamboozlement. At precisely six o'clock, he materializes, a short barrelly man dressed in a sleeveless robe of saffron and maroon. His scalp is shaven, and the only visible hair is a scanty black line above each hooded eye.

He bows in greeting while his young interpreter makes the introduction. Yeshi Dhonden, we are told, will examine a patient selected by a member of the staff. The diagnosis is unknown to Yeshi Dhonden as it is to us. The examination of the patient will take place in our presence, after which we will reconvene in the conference room where Yeshi Dhonden will discuss the case. We are further informed that for the past two hours Yeshi Dhonden has purified himself by bathing, fasting, and prayer. I, having breakfasted well, performed only the most desultory of ablutions, and given no thought at all to my soul, glance furtively at my fellows. Suddenly we seem a soiled, uncouth lot.

The patient had been awakened early, and told that she was to be examined by a foreign doctor, and had been asked to produce a fresh specimen of urine, so when we enter her room, the woman shows no surprise. She has long ago taken on that mixture of compliance and resignation that is the facies of chronic illness. This was to be but another in the endless series of tests and examinations. Yeshi Dhonden steps to the bedside while the rest stand apart watching. For a long time he gazes at the woman, favouring no part of her body with his eyes, but seeming to fix his glance at a place just above her supine form. I, too, study her. No physical sign nor obvious symptom gives a clue to the nature of her disease.

At last he takes her hand, raising it in both of his own. Now he bends over the bed in a kind of crouching stance, his head drawn down into the collar of his robe. His eyes are closed as he feels for her pulse. In a moment he has found the spot, and for the next half hour he remains thus, suspended above the patient like some exotic golden bird with folded wings, holding the pulse of the woman beneath his fingers, cradling her hand in his. All the power of the man seems to have been drawn down into this one purpose. It is palpation of the pulse raised to the state of ritual. From the foot of the bed where I stand, it is though he and the patient have entered a very special place of isolation, of apartness about which a vacancy hovers, and across which no violation is possible. After a moment the woman rests back upon her pillow. From time to time, she raises her head to look at the strange figure above her, then sinks back once more. I cannot see their hands joined in a correspondence that is exclusive, intimate, his fingertips receiving the voice of her sick body through the rhythm and throb she offers at her wrist. All at once I am envious – not of him, not of Yeshi Dhonden for his gift of beauty and holiness, but of her. I want to be held like that, touched so, *received*. And I know that I, who have palpated a hundred thousand pulses, have not felt a single one.

At last Yeshi Dhonden straightens, gently places the woman's hand upon the bed, and steps back. The interpreter produces a small wooden bowl and two sticks. Yeshi Dhonden pours a portion of the urine specimen into the bowl, and proceeds to whip the liquid with two sticks. This he does for several minutes until a foam is raised. Then, bowing above the bowl, he inhales the odor three times. He sets down the bowl, and turns to leave. All this while, he has not uttered a single word. As he nears the door, the woman raises her head and calls out to him in a voice at once urgent and serene. "Thank you, doctor," she says, and touches with her other hand the place he had held on her wrist as though to recapture something that had visited there. Yeshi Dhonden turns back for a moment to gaze at her, then steps into the corridor. Rounds are at an end.

We are seated once more in the conference room. Yeshi Dhonden speaks now for the first time, in soft Tibetan sounds that I have never heard before. He has barely begun when the young interpreter begins to translate, the two voices continuing in tandem – a bilingual fugue, the one chasing the other. It is like the chanting of monks. He speaks of winds coursing through the body of the woman, currents that break against barriers, eddying. These vortices are in her blood, he says. The last spendings of an imperfect heart. Between the chambers of her heart, long, long before she was born, a wind had come and blown open a deep gate that must never be opened. Through it charge the full waters of her river, as the mountain stream cascades in the spring-time, battering, knocking loose the land, and flooding her breath. Thus he speaks, and is silent. "May we now have the diagnosis?" a professor asks.

The host of these rounds, the man who knows, answers.

"Congenital heart disease," he says. "Interventricular septal defect, with resultant heart failure."

A gateway in the heart, I think, that must not be opened. Through it charge the full waters that flood her breath. So! Here is the doctor listening to the sounds of her body to which the rest of us are deaf.

Anatomised Bodies

"The Church says: the body is a sin.
Science says: the body is a machine.
Advertising says: The body is a business.
The body says: I am a fiesta."
(Galeano, 1997, p. 133)

Bodies

It may at first glance seem that our bodies are just bodies. We all have one, so what are they? How exactly do we define them? Our bodies are complex, and the business of explaining them is far from straightforward and easy.

For thousands of years before the arrival of the European Renaissance (and Vesalius along with it), people understood that they consisted of two parts – an eternal soul and the physical body that temporarily housed it during its human lifetime. It was then inconceivable to think of a person's body apart from its soul (Sawday, 1995). Everyone knew that when they died, their soul would depart this world, leaving their physical corpse behind it; just as somebody vacates a house that they have finished living in. It was therefore pretty obvious that a living person's body and their corpse were two quite different things.

The 16th and 17th centuries in Europe fostered the development of an emerging belief in the value of experimental and mathematical evidence to describe physical phenomena (including human anatomy). This new and more secular way of thinking had much going for it, although it was not equipped to explain the subtle, non-physical (spiritual) aspects of life. This soon led to a pragmatic, expertise-based division of responsibility for overseeing people's knowledge of their bodies. Simply put, the physical body form and its secular description were assigned to the domain of Science, while the nonphysical soul side of things remained with the Church and theologians.

This agreed-upon sharing out of roles made it possible for both parties to move on and do the work they were best qualified to do, without having to capitulate to each other's ways of thinking. It did not, however, conclusively sort out the question of what a human person's body actually is. One that is alive, breathing, and is, it would seem, still animated by some sort of life energy force or soul.

> "Talking about 'the body' and even 'your body' presupposes that a body is something easily defined, that there's something consistent about it through time. But think about your own body for a moment – is it that easy? Is your body actually the physical object you think it is right now? Does it change depending on who you are with? … Is your body somehow the embodiment of your own experiences, changing over time?" *(Roberts, 2021)*

Every human life is contingent on having a living body. We all have one. There are similarities between them, yet everyone's body is unique to them, irreplaceable, and priceless. Our bodies are naturally whole. They come in one piece, but, when you cut them open and anatomically dissect them, they appear to be formed from lots of different parts. The body, whatever we may think it is, is also incredibly hard to pin down and describe as it's constantly changing and moving, from the moment of its conception through to its death. The body you had as a child, for instance, looked quite different to the way it looks now, and maybe last year, even though it was-and-is the same body.

Our world's literature and art shows that people's bodies have been thought about, experienced, examined, and described from many different angles, all of which reflect the different kinds of investigative light (e.g., philosophical, methodological, technical) that has been shone on them at a specific time and place in the world's history. Each beam of light illuminates certain aspects (cf., mirrored disco ball facets) of the body's unfurling wholeness that we may previously have been unaware of, or known very little about. The wider the beam of light we individually and collectively shine on it, the more we can see what it truly is.

The ways we understand our bodies' structure depends on the ways 'the body' has been conceptualised, experienced, observed, illustrated and described *by people*. Little wonder that there's not just one or two, but many ways of defining what it is.[7] Those that are most relevant to this book include:

- Something whole that functions as an organised unit
- A material object that has physical existence and extension in space
- A mass of something that is perceptible to the sense of touch
- A person
- A corpse
- The complete physical or mortal form of a person, in contrast to their soul body
- The entire assemblage of parts, organs, and tissues that constitutes a person's material body
- The main, central, or principal parts, as distinguished from subordinate or less important parts, of a person's material body.

7 "body, n." *OED Online*, Oxford University Press, September 2020, www.oed.com/view/Entry/20934. Accessed 8 September 2020.

Anatomists

Anatomists are people who professionally describe the body's structural configuration. Nowadays, most – though not all – anatomists are scientists. Just like everyone else, they have a number of ways of finding-out-about and making sense of this complicated subject. As a result, there are now several branches of the anatomy profession, each of which sheds light on certain facets of the body's structural makeup (see Table 3.1). Their distinct yet interconnected ways of working help them collectively generate far richer, more extensive, and more comprehensive sets of anatomical information than would otherwise be possible (i.e., if they separately described it).

**Table 3.1
Branches of the
anatomy profession**

Each branch of the anatomy profession has a particular way of explaining the body's structure. For example, *gross anatomy* (also known as *macroscopic anatomy*) studies parts of the body that can ordinarily be seen with the naked eye. *Microscopic anatomy* instead examines much tinier parts of the body (e.g., cells, protein fibres) that can only be seen through a microscope.

GROSS ANATOMY Study of body's macroscopic structure	**Surface anatomy**	Study of external body features
	Systemic anatomy	Study of body structure from an organ systems perspective
	Regional anatomy	Study of body structure from a regional perspective
	Clinical anatomy	Study of anatomy relevant to clinical practice
	Surgical anatomy	Study of body structures relevant to surgeons
MICROSCOPIC ANATOMY Study of body's microscopic structure	**Organology**	Study of organs
	Histology	Study of tissues
	Cytology	Study of cellular structure
	Structural biology	Study of bio-molecular structure
RADIOLOGICAL ANATOMY	Study of body structure using X-rays and other imaging technology	
DEVELOPMENTAL ANATOMY	Study of structural changes from conception to birth	
BIOLOGICAL (OR PHYSICAL) ANTHROPOLOGY	Study of human biological variation and evolution	
COMPARATIVE ANATOMY	Study of similarity and differences between human and animal anatomy	
INTEGRATIVE ANATOMY	Study of body structure from a broad, transdisciplinary perspective	

By definition, anatomists *anatomise* the body. They *dissect* it, or cut it up, so that they can study the position, structure, and structural relations of its seemingly distinct parts. The anatomisation process happens in two main ways, although many people are only aware of the one that involves an anatomist wielding a sharp scalpel.

The first, and maybe more important one, occurs on an abstract level. Unless you're specifically aware of it, this intellectual trimming of how the body is envisaged is easily missed. In their naturally whole condition, our living bodies have a mindbogglingly complex structural form that, in theory, we are unlikely to ever fully understand (Heidegger, 1977).[8] In spite of this philosophical hiccup, there is still much to be gained by learning as much as we possibly can about them with the resources that are available to us. One way of doing this is to *academically dissect* the body, hypothetically reducing it into some smaller, more mentally manageable segments. This has meant, for example, regarding the body as a depersonalised and scientifically quantifiable physical object. This theoretical approach has in turn made it possible to conceptually equate a person's body with a human corpse. It has also allowed the body to be conveniently portrayed as a mechanistic, reconstituted assemblage of its (ostensibly) most important parts.

The second, and better known, type of anatomisation happens when anatomists *physically dissect* the body in order to visually reveal the position, structure, and relations of the parts it seems to consist of – including, for example, its lungs, tongue, and thyroid gland. To do this, they cut through the skin, then progressively separate the things that are stacked, each on top of the other, beneath it, until they have exposed the section they want to examine. Contrary to popular belief, most of the work is done with a blunt instrument (often the anatomist's fingers), and involves relatively little use of a sharp cutting blade.

Both types of dissection have invaluably enabled anatomists to examine and describe the body's structure in ways that people's

8   Heidegger (1889–1976), an enigmatic German philosopher, explained that the process of academic inquiry is essentially reductive, so can only ever apprehend part of something that is fundamentally much larger (1977). Viewed this way, anatomy researchers are equipped to study and describe (reveal) certain aspects of the body's structure. They are also inevitably (and possibly unknowingly) unequipped and unable to see or describe some other, potentially knowable aspects of it. These unseen (concealed) aspects may instead be attended to by, for example, anthropologists or artists.

minds can generally cope with. Dissection deconstructs the body so we can understand it. It literally and figuratively breaks it down into a host of separate, more mentally digestible, body parts.

The anatomy profession at large has already identified thousands of variously sized parts and particles that contribute to the body's structural form and will doubtless discover many more as our technical ability to see them continues to improve. Keeping track of these many different items has necessitated the development of a clear-cut conceptual framework that allows anatomists (and interested others) to name, describe, classify, and or distinguish between them all (see Table 3.2).

ORGANISM	A whole and alive person's body
ORGAN SYSTEM	A group of organs that work together to perform a particular set of body functions (e.g., muscular system)
ORGAN	A body part that performs a specific function (e.g., a muscle)
TISSUE	A group of cells that have a similar structure and function together as a unit (e.g., muscle tissue)
CELL	The smallest biological unit (e.g., a muscle cell)

Explaining body movement

Scientists have long been interested in finding out how our bodies move. As you might expect, their answers depend on how they anatomically visualise the body's structure. Different understandings about its structure will inevitably result in different explanations about its movement functioning. This is illustrated in the development of the following two movement models (i.e., ways of theoretically describing how the body moves), each of which embodies a different set of assumptions about our bodies' structural conformation. One of them, which has been around for several centuries, relates to the body's organ (muscle and bone) level of structure. The other has just emerged during the past few decades. It is premised on a more holistic understanding of the body form that enables it to consider the body's cellular through to organismic levels of movement activity.

(1) Biomechanical movement model

The first model was originally devised by Giovanni Alfonso Borelli (1608–1679), an Italian physiologist and mathematician. He compared the body's method of movement to a lever machine system, in which the application of mechanical force (*effort*) causes two rigid bars (*levers*) to move in relation to each other around a fixed point, or *fulcrum*. Levers amplify the force applied to an object. They are generally used to help lift a heavy load, or to move a load further or faster, with a minimal amount of energy (effort) input.

From this traditional *biomechanical*[9] viewpoint, the body's bones are likened to levers that pivot around the joint (fulcrum) between them. The force generated by a contracting muscle pulls (via its tendon) on the adjoining bone, causing it, and anything it might be carrying (*load*), to move in an arc through the space that surrounds them (see Figure 3.1).

The relative positional arrangement of a lever system's effort, load, and fulcrum parts (i.e., muscle, bone, and joint) affects the body's performance of a particular type of movement task. One type of lever system can, for example, help provide the power to shift a heavy rock, which might otherwise be impossible to move. Another might give a ballerina's foot the strength it needs to dance on the tips of its toes. And a different one may enable a major league power pitcher deliver a 105 miles per hour (170 km/h) fastball.

9 Biomechanics (or biological mechanics) applies the laws of classical mechanics to studying the structure and movement of biological systems, including anatomised human bodies.

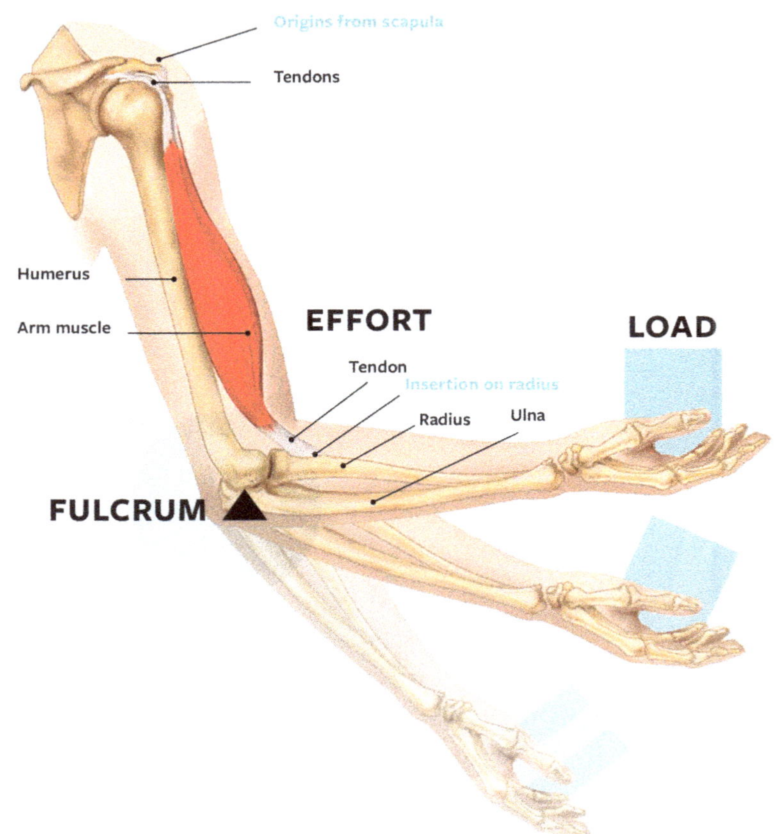

(2) Biotensegrity movement model

In the second type of movement model, the body is seen as being a *cohesive whole* structure rather than a collection of distinct (anatomised) musculo-skeletal *body parts* (i.e., muscles, bones, tendons, ligaments, and joints). This of course means that the body's movement is explained by a different set of theoretical principles.[10]

Richard Buckminster Fuller (1895–1983) was an American architect and systems theorist who coined the term *tensegrity* – a linguistic portmanteau of *tensional integrity* – to describe a type

10 The architectural theory that relates to this type of body form was inspired by the work of Kenneth Snelson (1927–2016), an American sculptor and photographer, and were subsequently explicated by his compatriot and professor, Richard Buckminster Fuller.

of structural system that is made from a set of solid struts (*intermittent compression elements*) that appear to float within a grid of taut cables (*continuous tension elements*) (see Figure 3.2). The struts don't physically touch each other as they are suspended and held in place by the tensional pull that continuously exists throughout the network of cables. The three-dimensional form and functioning of a tensegrity system structure depends on the balance of push and pull forces that exists within it at a particular moment in time. A tensegrity system's innate wholeness means that any force that is applied to it is automatically dispersed throughout the entire system. The current condition of each part of it affects all of the others. A push on one of the struts will in this way alter the balance and shape of the whole system structure, as will a tightening, or a lengthening, of one of the cables. The efficiency of their design means that tensegrity structures are light in weight, strong, and stable. They can change and resume their shape freely, with only a small outlay of energy.

Biotensegrity is a relatively new way of thinking about bodies and movement. It applies the principles of tensegrity to *all* types of biological structures – including, for example, people's bodies. The word *biotensegrity*, a blending of *biological* and *tensegrity*, was devised in the 1980s by Stephen M. Levin, an American orthopaedic surgeon and systems biologist. He realised that people's bodies are *not* like lever machines and *do not* obey the 17th century laws of classical mechanics. People's bodies are not built from a selection of anatomised body parts. In reality, they are naturally whole, coherently organised, multi-level (as in Table 3.2), living systems structures. The ways bodies move are "chaotic, non-linear, complex and unpredictable" (Levin, 2006, p. 79) – i.e., they are governed by laws of nature rather than those of classical mechanics.

From a biotensegrity perspective, the symmetry, stability, and strength of a person's body depends on the moment-by-moment

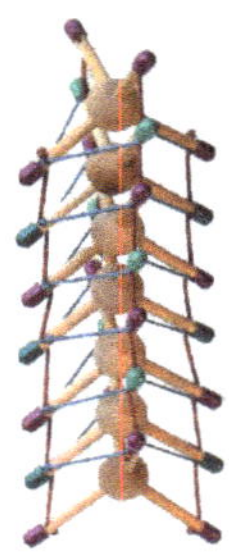

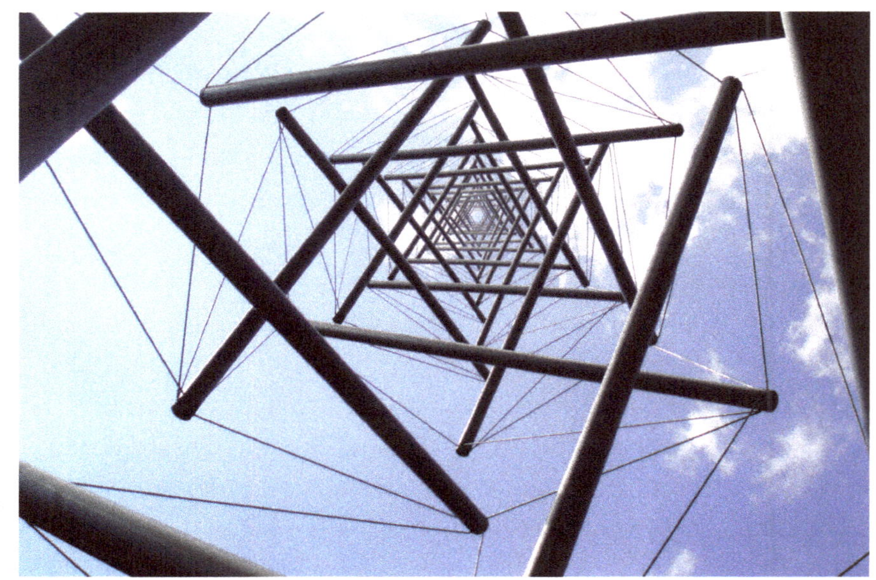

**Figure 3.2
Tensegrity and biotensegrity
structural systems.**

The photograph on the right shows
Kenneth Snelson's famous 'Needle
Tower' sculpture, in which a group
of solid struts are physically held in
place, supported by, and appear to
float within a grid of continuously
tensioned cables. The architectural
integrity of the entire tower
structure primarily depends on
tension held within the latticework
of cables, rather than the physical
strength of the rods themselves.
This architectural principle may be
applied to our understanding of
all biological structures (including,
but not only, bacteria, cells, and
animals' bodies) – hence the word
biotensegrity. The picture on the
left shows a model of the human
spine that was created by the artist
Tom Flemons. This wood and cord
model illustrates the biotensegrity
principle, in that the human back's
relatively solid wood 'vertebral
bones' are suspended by, and
move within, a web of continuously
tensioned 'soft tissue' cables.
This way of explaining the human
back's spinal structure differs from
its conventional biomechanical
depiction as a column of bones
that are physically stacked and
balanced one upon the other – an
idea that has now been shown to
be architecturally impossible in
a whole and constantly moving
living body. (To find out more, see
http://kennethsnelson.net/ and
https://intensiondesigns.ca/about/)

balance of push and pull forces that are distributed all the way through its entire fascia-, muscle-, and-bone-containing structure, not just the physical strength of some of its muscles, bones, ligaments, and tendons. From a biotensegrity perspective, a person's body movement results from an energy efficient cascade of changes in the geometric shape and position of one anatomical place within it in relation to another. It is, in this sense, a whole-body response that is driven by the body's structure rather than just its brain (Scarr, 2014). As a result, a shattered bone, a weak muscle, a surgical mesh implant, or wearing high heeled shoes (for instance) could alter the *entire* body structure and affect the way its organs, tissues, and cell contents all work – not just a small localised area of it.

> "Biology is not constrained by the laws of classical
> mechanics and, if there is to be a genuine understanding
> of its functions, an organism must always be considered
> in its entirety with each 'part' related to the whole."
> *(Scarr, 2014, p. 41)*

Both of these ways of modelling how our bodies move (i.e., biomechanical and biotensegrity) are based on a particular-yet-different understanding of the body's structural makeup. One involves a body that has been anatomised into discrete *parts* (i.e., bones, joints, ligaments, muscles and tendons). The other theoretically relates to a unified *whole*, multi-level (i.e., cell, tissue, organ, organ system, organism) and fascia-containing body construct. Each way of conceptualising the body's structure is valuable in helping us understand several different things about the body's movement functioning, but neither has the capacity to fully explain everything that really happens. Their different fields of vision mean we can choose to regard them as co-existing alongside, competing with, or complementary to each other. As a clinician, I personally find it helpful to combine the information contained in both of them, and hopefully develop a wider, and more richly nuanced understanding of the subject.

The biomechanical model, with its focus on local cause and effect, has regularly been used by doctors, physiotherapists, and sports trainers (for example) to help with their management of *musculoskeletal body problems*. This model's concepts have also played a central role in the development of many medical devices, such as artificial limbs, prosthetic hip and knee joints, replacement teeth, and the stents used to repair damaged arteries. In contrast, the biotensegrity model is still fairly new, and has yet to be widely applied in the medical world. Despite this, it has already revealed its potential to greatly improve our understanding of our bodies' architecture and movement mechanisms.

Fascia

Finding fascia

You would be far from alone if you don't know what fascia is.[11] For the first twenty years of my professional life as a physiotherapist in New Zealand, I didn't either. I was vaguely aware of, but knew almost nothing about, the *fascia lata* and *thoracolumbar fascia* (sheets of dense tissue in the thigh and low back) and *tensor fasciae latae* (a small muscle in the thigh). Fascia by itself was not expressly mentioned in our early 1970s student lectures or textbooks. It was not considered when treating our patients. It was not discussed with my health professional colleagues, nor at any seminars or conferences I attended. It was as if it did not exist, yet, as I've since learned, fascia is an extremely important part of our bodies.

I first became interested in fascia when I was trying to find a cure for my own neck and back pain, in the early 1980s. The then-routine forms of treatment – bed rest, foam collars, hot packs, joint mobilisation, exercises, and pills – usually helped in the short term, but weren't providing the long-lasting relief I wanted. A by-chance meeting with a visiting Rolfer®[12] led to my receiving a short series of her fascia-relating bodywork treatments. Which, much to my surprise, soon healed my old pain problems for good.

11 Fascia is pronounced *fash-ee-uh*.

12 Licensed Rolfing® Structural Integration practitioner.

This encounter alerted me to the existence of fascia, and activated my sense that it might perhaps be important. Since then, I have been lucky to receive, study, and sometimes teach others about several types of fascia-relating bodywork treatment – including the Upledger and the Milne methods of craniosacral therapy, and John Barnes's myofascial release therapy.

As a physiotherapist, I was extremely interested in my patients' and other practitioners' apparent successes with these ways of working, especially when they seemed to help ease some health problems that, in my experience, were not then normally treated with hands-on-body (manual) therapy. It seemed that many medical conditions including, for example, asthma, autism, birth injuries in babies, chronic pain, digestive problems, endocrine imbalances, gynaecological conditions, headaches, head injuries, hypertension, learning disorders, musculoskeletal injuries, neurological problems, post-natal depression, post-traumatic stress disorder, problematic scars, painful sinuses, and impacted teeth might possibly be helped with manual techniques – in conjunction with regular medical attention.

Even though most of my patients seemed to benefit from their fascia-relating bodywork treatments, I was concerned by my inability to explain why this work seemed to be helping them in the scientific terms valued by my profession. I was keen to introduce this new type of treatment to my professional community, but knew I first needed to learn a lot more about it, and fascia. I did this by returning to university as a 'mature student,' and studying a wide variety of subjects – including anatomy, anthropology, medical history, and public health – and developed the 'big-picture,' transdisciplinary viewpoint I now use in my teaching and writing (see footnote 1, page xii).

A brief history of fascia

Fascia is a non-specific anatomical term that broadly refers to the body's soft connective tissue parts. *Fascia* is probably a Latinised version of an ancient Greek word ταινία (*taenia*) (Adstrum & Nicholson, 2019). In the days of ancient Greece and Rome, both of these words generally related to thin, strip-like objects, such as bandages, building surfaces, headbands, sashes, ribbons, strips of land, strips of cloud, tape-worms, and certain types of long, thin fish.[13] These days, *fascia* is also applied to the naming of, for example, the flat surface on an advertising sign, a band of colour on a bird's plumage, a row of holes on a seashell, the removable front face surface of a mobile phone, and even the web of subtle connections that exist between people and the world they live in.[14]

The word *fascia* appears to have entered English language medical writing in anatomist Helkiah Crooke's (1615 & 1651) description of the body's "almost infinite" number of membranes (Adstrum & Nicholson, 2019). With time, his anatomical use of this term was picked up and expanded upon by others. Yet, for most of the next 200 years, this term was more often than not used in the names of surgical bandages, rather than body tissue – e.g., *fascia spiralis* (a spiral roller bandage) and *fascia tortilis* (a name for a tourniquet).

Fascia came to the fore during the 19th and 20th centuries, when advances in research technology made it much more visible to anatomists than it had been in the past. Newly developed cadaver and tissue preservation methods prevented the body's soft tissues from decaying (which they naturally do fairly quickly), allowing them to remain visible and be examined in detail. The tissue-preserving fluids often contained chemicals (e.g., alcohol, formaldehyde) that, along with lengthy exposures to air in the dissection laboratory, tended to dry out and condense the dead body's fascia. This was a mixed blessing. On one hand,

13 This word is still used by anatomists to refer to some flat bands of tissue in the colon (*taeniae ccli*) and in the brain (*taenia thalami* and *taenia of the 4th ventricle*).

14 As in Ashley Donielle Murray's *Fascia* (2009), a compilation of vignettes that highlights some of the intangible threads of familial and community connection that contributed to the fabric of her southern American childhood.

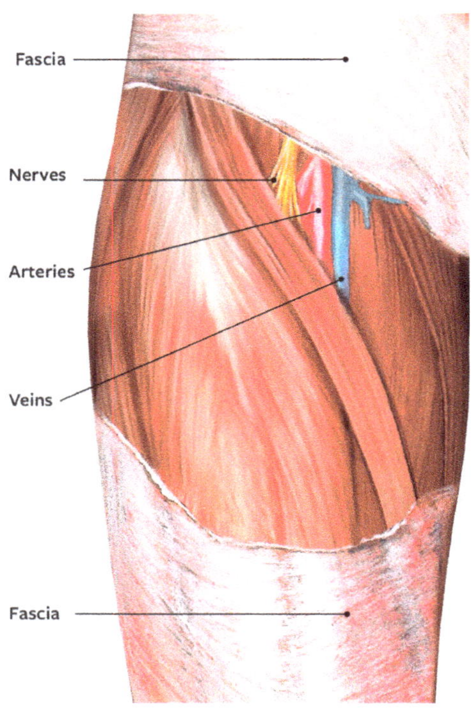

Figure 4.1
Before and after cleaning

This is an artist's rendition that shows what the surface layer of trunk and thigh muscles, nerves (yellow), arteries (red) and veins (blue) look like before and after the outer layer of gauzy white fascia that normally covers them has been 'cleaned' away (removed) during the anatomical dissection process.

it was now easy to see the sheets of the unnaturally dehydrated and dense tissue – a factor that contributed to the anatomical discovery of many new sections of fascia (*fasciae*) (Warwick & Williams, 1973). On the other, the dried out fascial tissue, no longer plumped full of water, was unnaturally thick and opaque and hid pretty much everything it covered. It became a nuisance for the anatomists who were no longer able to see through it to examine anything else, such as muscles, blood vessels, and internal organs. This led to fascia being routinely *cleaned* away (removed and discarded) in the dissection lab (see Figure 4.1), and then being largely forgotten about by many anatomists, by their students – who later became health practitioners, health researchers, health educators, and health writers – and by the public at large, most of whom probably hadn't heard of it in the first place.

Around about the first decade of the 21st century, this state of affairs began to change. People from many walks of life had begun talking about fascia *as if* it might be something important. Fascia was now being studied by many types of researchers, including, but not mostly (as in the past), anatomists and surgeons. Their wide-ranging interests and the varied nature of their clinical and scientific work soon revealed that, between them all, they had some quite different ideas about what the word *fascia* meant to them. Was it a dissectible piece of tissue? The tissue that made up the dissectible pieces of fascia? Or a whole body-pervading web of a soft tissue substance that assumed a variety of function-related textures and forms?

A past lack of clear definition meant *fascia* was now being interpreted to mean any or all three of these things – a type of body tissue, a type of dissectible body part, and a type of body system. This ambiguity was coupled with disparities in the way fascia was being portrayed in medical dictionaries, anatomy textbooks, scientific research reports, in different countries, and in different clinical professions. Everyone had their own ideas about what fascia was, and, just like the six blind scholars who described an elephant, sort of assumed that everyone else thought about it in the same way. The problem was that they didn't.

Once they realised what was happening, alarm bells rang within the emerging fascia research community. Their members were rightly concerned that erratic use of this word to refer to any of several types of body part was interfering with people's understanding of, and communication about, fascia (Adstrum et al., 2017). For them all – be they health care professionals, anatomists, or other types of scientists – it is vital that every anatomical term (including *fascia*) explicitly relates to *one and the same* type of body part. If it doesn't, any ambiguity needs to be fixed, and fixed fast. Fortunately the fascia research community was able to do this by devising two new anatomical terms – a *fascia*, and the *fascial system* (see Table 4.1). With any luck, this simple measure would help people say what they meant when they talked about fascia.

Table 4.1
Contemporary language of fascia

Until recently, the word *fascia* was used to convey several overlapping yet different sets of anatomical meaning. This newly defined set of terms is now helping people distinguish between these different aspects of fascia (i.e., tissue, organ, organ system).

TERM	GENERAL MEANING	FORMAL DEFINITION
Fascia	All of the body's soft connective tissue parts	A non-specific word that anatomists apply to "sheaths, sheets or other dissectible masses of connective tissue that are large enough to be visible to the unaided eye as well as the tissue from which they are composed" (Standring, 2016b, p. 41).
Fascial tissue	Soft connective tissue	Connective tissue proper.
A fascia (plural, fasciae)	A distinct and dissectible piece of fascial tissue	"A sheath, a sheet or any number of dissectible aggregations of connective tissue that forms beneath the skin to attach, enclose, separate muscles and other internal organs" (Stecco & Schleip, 2016, p. 139).
The fascial system	A body-pervading web of fascial tissue	"The three-dimensional continuum of soft, collagen containing loose and dense fibrous connective tissues that permeate the body. It incorporates elements such as adipose tissue, adventitiae and neurovascular sheaths, aponeuroses, deep and superficial fasciae, epineurium, joint capsules, ligaments, membranes, meninges, myofascial expansions, periostea, retinacula, septa, tendons, visceral fasciae, and all the intramuscular and intermuscular connective tissues including endo-/peri-/epimysium. The fascial system surrounds, interweaves between, and interpenetrates all organs, muscles, bones and nerve fibers, endowing the body with a functional structure, and providing an environment that enables all body systems to operate in an integrated manner" (Adstrum et al., 2017, p. 175; & Stecco et al., 2018, p. 354).

Another tipping point?

To put it mildly, there has been a strong revival of interest in fascia during the past two decades. This is evident, for example, in the steep growth in the number of fascia-relating reports being published in peer-reviewed journals, in the staging of several major international Fascia Research Congresses, and many more fascia-focused symposia. It can also be seen in a recent upsurge of new books about fascia and fascial therapies, and an unprecedented level of media interest – including television documentaries, webinars, and audiovisual learning resources. Interestingly, all of this has been accompanied by a staggering growth in the number of Google keyword results for *fascia* – i.e., the number of Internet webpages that mention this particular word.[15] These have, according to my records, risen from around 14,000 in October 2008, to 36 million in October 2011, to more than 92 million now (in July 2021).[16] Lots and lots of people are now interested in fascia – not just anatomists and surgeons. It also appears that their (including the clinical anatomy profession's) present understandings of it may have moved on from the ways it was known in the 20th century.

Clinical Anatomy (CA) is a well-respected international anatomy journal that facilitates the exchange of reliable, up-to-date information between anatomists, clinicians, and anatomy educators. Its readership includes anatomists, many types of health-related professionals (including surgeons, physicians, dentists, physiotherapists, medical imaging specialists, pathologists), medical educators, medical residents, and health science students.

Every year, CA's editorial team produces eight peer-reviewed journal issues that keep their readers well-informed about their ever-changing professional landscape. In keeping with normal practice, CA is served by an editorial advisory board, whose

15 Some of which do not relate to the anatomical meaning of this term.

16 While Google search result numbers are an approximation, and result numbers for the same search keyword may fluctuate up or down slightly due to a number of factors, the overall trend for *fascia* has been a strongly upward one.

tasks include identifying topics for special issues (which they may be invited to guest edit). Several of CA's forty-four editorial board members have links to the fascia research community, so (by around 2015) they were well aware that fascia was attracting an extraordinary amount of interdisciplinary attention. Maybe this would be something interesting and useful for their journal's readers to know about?

After this idea had been duly discussed by the editorial team, a decision was made to go ahead and compile a special issue that featured fascia. A guest editor was appointed, and a range of fascia researchers were invited to report on their work. Volume 32, Issue 7, CA's Special Issue on Fascia, was published online on the 9th of September, 2019, and the 110-page-long printed version was mailed the following week. Some of the several topics covered included the history of fascia, contractile properties of fascia, myofascial chains, fascial entrapment neuropathy, and the novel concept of fasciatomes.

The editorial, penned by CA's editor-in-chief notably explains that this special issue discusses "an underrepresented part of the human frame, the fascia" (Tubbs, 2019, p. 861). His text draws on an observation attributed to Philipp Melanchthon, a highly influential 16th century German Lutheran scholar, that says, "It is shameful for man to rest in ignorance of the structure of his own body, especially when the knowledge of it mainly conduces to his welfare, and directs his application of his own powers."

Melanchthon (1497–1560) lived in Europe at the same time as Andreas Vesalius, and was a great fan of Vesalius's new scientific approach to anatomy research. During this historical period people generally accepted that they and their bodies were made by a heavenly Creator. For Melanchthon, anatomy was extremely important because of the theological linkages between the body, the soul, and Christian morality. Anatomy described something designed by the Creator, and people were morally bound to use this knowledge to help them take the best possible care of their (own and each other's) bodies. It would be *shameful* (i.e., morally despicable) for them to do otherwise.

All of this meant that it was really important that anatomists described the body as accurately as possible. For Melanchthon, this meant scientifically, just like Vesalius was then doing – i.e., untainted by the religious dogma that had perpetuated Galen's anatomy ideas for nearly 1500 years. Scientifically improving the quality of anatomical knowledge would, from Melanchthon's point of view, lessen people's ignorance of the structure of their own bodies, and enable them to look after them properly. That is to say, without any illogical religious nonsense! Which he, as a Protestant, believed they were morally bound to do.

A big part of what made Melanchthon remarkable was that he didn't just sit around and talk about these sorts of things. He rolled up his sleeves and used his considerable academic authority to reorganise the ways anatomy and medicine were taught in Germany's Protestant universities. Between them, Melanchthon and his friend Vesalius succeeded in advancing the way people are able to think about human anatomy and improving their health.

The publication of CA's Special Issue on Fascia, together with the serious tone of its introductory editorial suggests that this journal's readers are being invited to update their understanding of fascia, so that it is perhaps more in tune with the ways fascia is being described in today's interdisciplinary research environment. This raises the possibility that the clinical anatomy profession may be experiencing another extremely important tipping point – one that is associated with a change in the way fascia and the body that contains it are recognised. Should this actually be happening, which it highly likely is, this could help facilitate a stepping forward in the ways we are all able to consider the body's (fascia-inclusive) anatomical structure, functioning, pathology, and health care.

Fascial Anatomy

Parts and wholes

Up until the late 20th century, fascia was usually only described by anatomists and surgeons. The nature of their day-to-day work meant they mostly saw it with their bare eyes (macroscopically) and, as a result, perceived it as a loosely defined collection of dissectible *body parts* (see Table 5.1).

Thinking about fascia as a group of dissectible body parts is definitely useful. It makes it possible for us to know what's what, and where exactly it is located inside the body. It helps us identify and distinguish between various sections of the body's three-dimensional continuum of fascial tissue. It helps us build a detailed map that charts the body's topographic features. Surgery, for example, would be terribly risky without this type of information. As would receiving an injection. Radiology and oncology reports couldn't be written, and researchers wouldn't be able to compare their findings. Anatomy and medical textbooks would be meaningless, and goodness knows how we might otherwise teach our trainee health practitioners. Even though this has been the main way of describing fascia in the past, it is not the only way fascia has been anatomically accounted for.

Table 5.1
Fascial body parts

Anatomists have traditionally described fascia in relation to three general layers of fascia, hundreds of pieces of fascia (fasciae), and a variable assortment of fascial body bits. Most of these fascial body parts are named for their physical appearance or location in the body. Some have also been eponymously named after an influential member of their profession (Adstrum, 2015).

	EXAMPLES	DESCRIPTION
LAYERS OF FASCIA	**Superficial fascia**	Layer of soft fibro-fatty tissue that covers most of the body just under the skin.
	Deep fascia	Layers of dense fibrous tissue that cover muscles.
	Visceral fascia	Internal column of fascia that lines the neck, chest, abdominal, and pelvic body cavities; and is wrapped around, and packed in-between, the organs inside them.
PIECES OF FASCIA	**Cribriform fascia (Hesselbach fascia)**	Sieve-like piece of fascia in the groin that has many tiny holes in it. From Latin *cribrum* (sieve). Eponymously named after Franz Hesselbach (1759–1816), a German anatomist and surgeon.
	Deltoid fascia	Fascia covering the deltoid muscle (a triangle-shaped muscle that covers the shoulder). Named after the Greek letter *delta* (Δ).
	Fascia lata	Large fascial sleeve encasing the thigh muscles. From Latin *lata* (broad).
	Plantar fascia	Thick layer of fascia covering muscles in the sole of the foot. From Latin *planta* (sole of foot).
	Renal fascia	Fascial envelope surrounding a kidney. From Latin *renes* (kidneys).
FASCIAL BODY BITS	**Epimysium**	Fascial sheath encasing a muscle.
	Epineurium	Fascial sheath encircling a nerve.
	Intermuscular septum	Fascial partition between two groups of muscles.
	Neurovascular sheath	Fascial sleeve encircling a nerve (or nerves) and its associated blood and lymph vessels.
	Organ capsule	Fascial sheath encasing an organ (e.g., kidney, eye).

Andrew Taylor Still (1828–1917) was an innovative, largely self-educated, American frontier medical doctor who perceived fascia quite differently to the ways it was then being construed (i.e., as a collection of dissectible body parts) in the anatomy and surgery literature. Dr. Still lived far away from any metropolitan medical schools that were equipped with professors, dissection laboratories, and libraries. This meant that his medical training was based on apprenticeship, rounded out by his own reading and research observations (which was not uncommon at that time in American history).

Dr. Still lived during a period when many people were questioning the safety and efficacy of the harsh drugs, sweating, purging, and blood-letting that were then routinely being used by the orthodox medical profession. The tragic deaths of three of his four young children from meningitis sealed his own disenchantment with these drastic, dangerous, expensive, and often completely ineffective forms of treatment. For him, the death of his children was an important turning point that prompted him to search for a better way of helping his patients recover their health. Many years of study and contemplation led to him developing a more natural, safer, and apparently more reliable system of medical care that he called osteopathy.

One of the key things that distinguished osteopathy from conventional medicine was the way it saw the body's structure. Dr. Still endorsed a holistic understanding of anatomy that explicitly related to the body's innate wholeness and aliveness *as well as* its anatomised parts. He compared the importance of knowing about both of them to describing a chicken's body. The chicken's body parts, he explained – including its head, gizzard, heart, and muscular system – "belong to the chicken," but the chicken would not be a chicken if any of them were missing. "They must all be present and pass roll call or we do not have a complete chicken" (1899, p. 17). If we want to understand the body properly, we definitely need to know about it from both angles. We need to know about its parts *and also* about its entirety.

Dr. Still wrote at length about fascia, emphasising the crucial role its tissue plays in unifying the body's structure and functioning from the moment of a person's conception through to the time they draw their last breath. In his words (1899), "The fascia is universal in man and equal in self to all other parts" (p. 163), and "I believe that more rich golden thought will appear to the mind's eye as the study of fascia is pursued than of any other division of the body" (pp. 22–23).

Osteopathy's principles and practices are grounded in the belief that:

- People are an amalgamation of body, mind, and spirit.
- People's bodies are naturally whole, so that everything in them is connected to and affected by everything else.
- The body's structure and function are mutually linked and influence each other.
- The body is able to regulate its own internal conditions (e.g., temperature, fluid balance, chemical levels) so it functions as well as it can.
- The body is able to heal itself and maintain its own health.

Osteopathy's treatments are therefore directed towards helping the whole person rather than just their physical disease symptoms (Lewis, 2012; Paulus, 2009 & 2013).

Fascial tissue

Fascial tissue is basically a gooey gel that contains several types of cells and a varying number of strengthening structural protein fibres in its body-pervading fabric (see Figure 5.1). It has not always been described this way, but this is what it's actually like in people's *whole and alive* bodies.

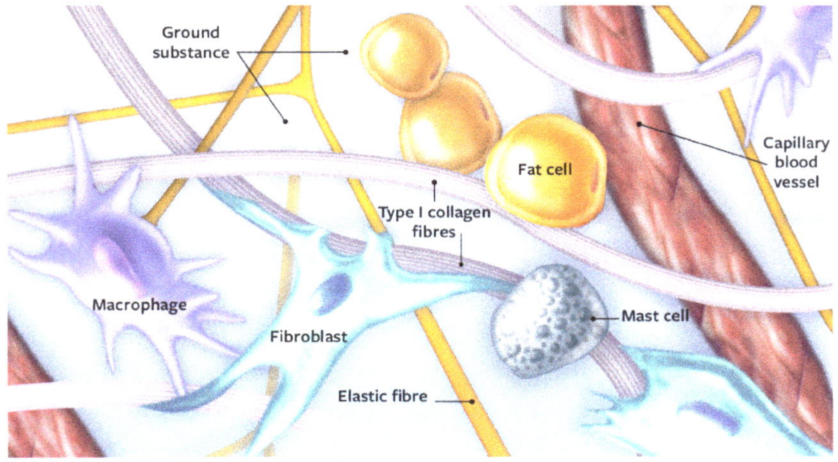

Figure 5.1
Fascial tissue

Fascial tissue contains a varying mix of cells and fibres in its ubiquitous ground substance. In some places, the fascial tissue is reinforced with many more Type I collagen fibres than are shown in this diagram, making it denser and stronger. These areas of denser tissue typically contain less, and fewer types of, cells – as most of the space is occupied with Type I collagen fibres. (Adapted from Marieb & Hoehn, 2019, Fig. 4.9, p. 160.)

Fascia's semi-solid ground substance is its most voluminous and traditionally least described tissue component. This is understandable because it is essentially just jellified water. At any one time, some parts of it will be more sticky than others. Some will be more liquidy and free-flowing (Benias et al., 2018). And some could be changing from one relatively glutinous or watery state to another (Pollack, 2001). When the gel's surface tension, or the membrane containing it in place, is artificially broken (e.g., by being physically pulled apart, or pierced with the tip of a scalpel) the gel immediately shatters into an open-weave mesh of flimsy threads. The shattered gel is often called areolar tissue (or loose connective tissue), because of the spaces (areas) between the threads. In its natural (living) condition, this varyingly viscous gel is normally transparent, and, unless you are using some state-of-the-art research tools (like those used, for instance, by Benias et al., 2018), seems to lack any definable features or shape. Fascia's gel substance is usually dried out, damaged, and or done away with by the processes of anatomy, histology, and surgery. It is artificially diminished and altered. It is not at all interesting to look at through an ordinary microscope. Not nearly as interesting as the fibres and cells that are embedded in it. It has accordingly received relatively little descriptive attention.

In many parts of the body, the fascia's gel substance is physically reinforced with some structural protein fibres. *Type I collagen,*[17] by far the most abundant type of fascial fibre, is white coloured and extremely strong. Fascial tissue is not (despite what many textbooks have implied) universally fortified with these fibres. They are only found in places where the tissue needs to be tough enough to withstand being stretched and pulled without tearing or breaking. *Elastin fibres* are, as their name suggests, elastic. Their presence permits the sections of fascia that contain them to stretch and recoil in step with the changing shape of the body part beneath them (e.g., a contracting-relaxing muscle).

Fascia also contains a variety of cells, whose being there fluctuates in accordance with the functional demands placed on its different sections of tissue at any given time. *Fibroblasts,* fascia's foremost cell type, are mainly responsible for secreting and maintaining the condition of gel and fibre matrix. Depending on its circumstances and requirements, fascial tissue may also contain some *adipocytes* (fat cells), and an occasional *macrophage* or *mast cell* from the body's immune defence team. Several other types of cell – including red blood cells, bacterial cells, white blood cells (e.g., lymphocytes, neutrophils), cancer cells, fungal cells – may at times be found in tissue that is injured or diseased.

From a histology point of view, fascia is now generally pigeon-holed as *connective tissue proper* (see Table 5.2). Its naturally intact gel substance pervades the entire body. In many places in the body, it forms into delicate sacs and membranes. In others, it is condensed into tough, collagen-dominant sheets, cords, bands, and ropes. Fascia accumulates between the body's

17 Type I collagen was the first of (so far) about 30 different types of collagen to be found in human bodies.

other parts (more about this in Chapter 7), seamlessly segueing from one functionally-modified form into another. Each specific variation helps make it possible for a particular section of its body-wide web of tissue to deal with the functional demands placed on it at any given moment in its body-owner's life.

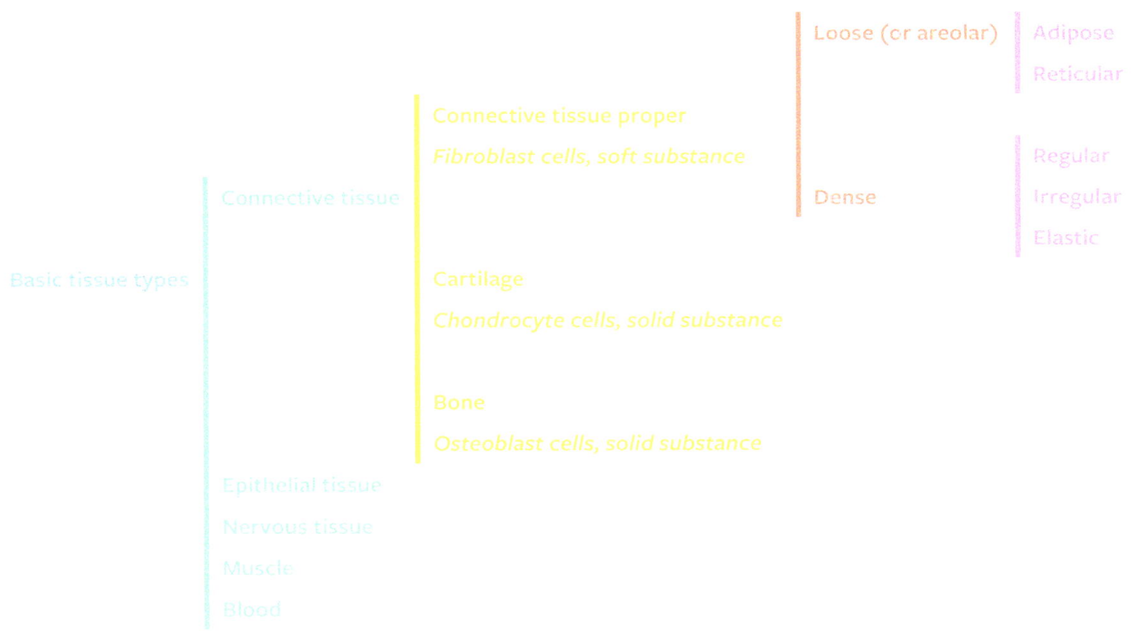

Fascia's qualities and functions

Fascia has a number of qualities (i.e., *how it is*) and functions (i.e., *what it does*) that are largely governed by the mix of cells, fibres and ground substance in its tissue. For most of the past 200 years, the only people who saw human fascia on a regular basis were anatomists and surgeons. This meant that their interest in *what it actually does* was restricted to the ways they experienced it in their work. As a result, fasciae were usually

**Table 5.2.
Classification of tissue**

Human tissue is categorised on the basis of its main type of cells, the relative solidity of the substance that may (or may not) surround them, and the organisation of their Type I collagen fibres (if they have them). Fascia's exact place in this schema has always been a bit vague and has largely depended on who wrote the textbook. On the whole, fascia is generally equated to connective tissue proper, or to one or more sub-categories of connective tissue proper.

considered to be made of a reasonably strong, yet basically inert kind of fibrous tissue that passively invests, contains, separates, covers, obscures, and fills in the gaps between the seemingly more highly developed and important body parts such as muscles, blood vessels, nerves, and visceral organs.

The recent surge of interdisciplinary research attention is generating lots of new information about fascia – including its qualities and functions (see Tables 5.3 & 5.4). This new knowledge is transforming the ways the body and its endless web of fascial tissue are being understood, cared for, and remedied in today's world. Fascia's relatively recent apperception as a three-dimensional continuum of tissue has made it possible for it to *additionally* be considered as the body's *medium of connection*. It joins everything else together – all of the body's cells, tissues, organs, organ systems. It unifies all the parts into a living body whole. It helps hold them all in place and protects each and all of them from harm. It powerfully enables them all to develop and grow. To function as they are meant to. To repair and heal. Fascia's ubiquity and interconnectedness allows every single part of the body to communicate and have dealings with every other part. It is, as some people say, fascianating stuff.

"There has been a paradigm shift in how fascia is known. The old way of describing fascia was someone opening up the body from the outside and showing all of the layers. We now know there are no layers and spaces. Everything is continuous. We now see the whole, vibrating fascial web." *(Professor Carol Davis, British Fascia Symposium, 2020)*

QUALITY	DESCRIPTION
Adaptive	Fascia has the ability to modify its gel-cells-fibre structure so that it can adapt to, recover from, and contribute to changes in its environment (e.g., aging, growth, hormonal fluctuations, metabolic demands, infection, tissue injury).
Anisotropic	Fascia's response to mechanical loading is directionally dependent. It behaves in differing ways when pulled from different directions (i.e., if you stretch it one way it closes, and if you stretch it the other way it opens). This is largely due to the directional alignment of its Type I collagen fibres (Stecco et al. 2009).
Bioelectromagnetic capacity	Fascia is capable of generating, conducting, and responding to energy phenomena (e.g., ions, electrical currents, electromagnetic fields). This is likely due (at least in part) to fascia's liquid crystalline molecular structure, its ability to become electrically polarised when it is stretched or compressed, and the movement of ion-containing fluids through its water- and electrolyte-rich ground substance (Oschman, 2012).
Complex	Fascia is constantly adapting and changing its structure. It is metabolically active and is constantly moving. Its three-dimensional, body pervading substance adopts a variety of forms in different parts of the body – including, membranes, sacs, sheets, tubes, sheaths, strands, bands, and layers within layers – all of which are seamlessly fitted together and stacked on top of each other. Its complexity has made it remarkably hard to concisely describe.
Continuous	Fascia is an uninterrupted and unbroken continuum of tissue that envelops and penetrates into each and every body part. This means that seemingly distinct body parts merge with each other and blend with their fascial surroundings. For example, the fascial substance of the gluteus maximus (buttock) muscle is continuous with the superficial layer of thoracolumbar fascia *and* with fascia lata in the thigh, and the latissimus dorsi muscle on the opposite side of the back. It also means that some so-called musculoskeletal problems may be linked to some tight fascia in the abdomen or thorax (and vice versa).

QUALITY	DESCRIPTION
Contractile	Some sections of fascia contain smooth muscle-like cells (myofibroblasts) that cause the nearby fascia, and muscles and joints it is associated with, to stiffen over a period of several minutes or longer (Schleip et al., 2019).
Elastic	Healthy fascial tissue is able to resume its normal shape after being stretched or compressed. This helps the body to harmlessly absorb physical shock, and to regain its original form after being stretched or compressed.
Healthy/unhealthy	Fascia is normally healthy though it can be adversely affected by infection, tumours, injury, postural misuse, inadequate nutrition, and dehydration (for instance), so may exhibit varying states of health and repair. Fascia may be also afflicted by fascia-related disorders such as compartment syndrome, Dupuytren's contracture, myofascial trigger points, plantar fasciitis, scleroderma, fibromyalgia, and rheumatoid arthritis. Malfunctioning fascia contributes to the development of congenital cleft lip and cleft palate, and varicose veins. Fascia is widely thought to play an important role in a diverse range of emotional, musculoskeletal, neurological, respiratory, and vascular health disorders.
Hydrated	Fascial (ground) substance normally contains lots of water, most of which has jellified around some large molecules (e.g., glycosaminoglycans, proteoglycans). The resulting gel provides fascia's ground substance with most of its volume, turgor (internal pressure), and resistance to compression (Young et al., 2014). This hydrated gel also enables the Type I collagen fibres to maintain sufficient distance from each other, which normally prevents them from sticking together in clumps. At any one time, some parts of the fascial ground substance gel will be more gelatinous than others, others will be more liquidy (Benias et al., 2018), and some others will be in the process of changing from one state to the other (Pollack, 2001). The more liquidy parts facilitate the free flow of nutrients, metabolites, cells, and information-signalling molecules through fascial tissue.

QUALITY	DESCRIPTION
Mobile	Fascia is normally mobile. It glides smoothly in some places, is anchored in others, and enables movement within and between the body's numerous parts. Some fasciae are more mobile than others. Unhealthy fascia is often associated with a decline in mobility and abnormal sticking together of body parts.
Omnipresent	Fascia is widespread and constantly encountered throughout the whole body. It has recently been estimated that fascia makes up approximately 17% of a person's body mass (Schleip & Stecco, 2021).[18]
Plastic	Plasticity is a property of solids that causes them to change permanently in size or shape when they are overstretched. This means that the structure and shape of a section of fascia can be permanently changed when it is subjected to a strong mechanical force – e.g., (negatively) following a severe ankle sprain injury, or (positively) with some manual therapy techniques.
Pliable	Healthy fascial tissue has a soft supple texture, is intrinsically flexible, and can be easily bent.
Sensitive	Fascial (ground) substance is richly endowed with sensory nerve endings, so is able to detect and respond to slight changes, signals, or influences within its environment. When healthy, fascia plays a significant part in sensing, and contributing to the coordination of, the relative position of body parts, posture, balance, motion, muscle tone, tissue stretch, autonomic tone and pain. Various fasciae are differently sensitive.
Somatoemotional capacity*	Is able to retain and to release stored memory of emotional injury events within its physical (somatic) substance. *This quality is widely acknowledged by bodywork clinicians, though it has yet to be scientifically tested and verified.*
Strong	Healthy fascial tissue is physically tough and strong, so has the capacity to withstand and transmit great force or pressure whilst maintaining its structural integrity. Some sections of fascia are much stronger, or more fragile, than others.

18   Schleip & Stecco's calculation was based on Tanaka & Kawamura's (1992) report about the composition of a statistically average Asian male body – i.e., aged between 20–50 (av. 35) years old, with a normal BMI (=22).

QUALITY	DESCRIPTION
Thixotropic	Fascia's ground substance is thixotropic, which means that it is able to change from a jelly-like solid to a more liquid solution (and vice versa). It tends to become more fluid/less viscous when it is stretched and heated (e.g., with exercise, or bodywork treatment). The reverse happens (i.e., it becomes more viscous) when the tissue is static or cold for lengthy periods of time.
Viscoelastic	Viscoelasticity is a property of materials (including fascia) that exhibit elastic *and* viscous characteristics when they are being physically deformed. The viscoelasticity of tissue varies with its physical condition (e.g., level of hydration, ionic content, pH) hence is likely to vary in different fasciae, and in different people.
Warm, squishy, and full of energy	In its natural condition (inside a living person's body) fascia feels warm and squishy to touch, due to its hydration and the liquidity of the fat contained within it. (Fat is usually solid in non-living tissue yet is liquid at body temperature, ~37 °C/98 °F.)

Fascia endows the body and all of its parts with their characteristic shape, and helps hold them all in their correct places and positions – hence its popular designation as the body's *organ of support* (Rolf, 1977), and the *organ of form* (Varela & Frenk, 1987). In this way, fascia, for example, "keeps our livers from falling out, our lungs and heart from exploding, and our intestines from falling down to the bottom of our pelvises" (Upledger, 2009, p. 24).

Type I collagen-reinforced fascial tissue is physically strong enough to bear considerable amounts of mechanical force without breaking. It helps anchor muscles to bones as well as to each other. It transmits the force generated by contracting muscle through its three-dimensional (epimuscular) surroundings. From a biotensegrity perspective, this collagen-strengthened fascia serves as the continuously tensioned web of *cables* that help suspend the bones (*struts*) in place and stabilise the joints between them. In this way, fascia serves as an energy-efficient tensegrity scaffold that architecturally enables all of the body's posture and movement activities.

Fascia's gel substance acts like a water-filled cushion that enables the energy efficient and gliding movement that normally occurs within and between the body's multitude of parts – including muscles, tendons, fasciae, and nerves. It serves as a spongy buffer that is interposed between all of these parts, permitting them to move freely without rubbing and being damaged. As a result, it may be thought of as the body's *medium of movement*.

The body's three-dimensional web of fascial substance houses, and is structurally continuous with, all of the body's fluid-conveying pipes and channels – including the blood and lymphatic vessels, capillaries, and interstitial fluid flows. In this way fascia physically supports and protects these important fluid transit routes. It helps keep them open and unobstructed so that the body's life-sustaining fluids, along with their important cargoes of oxygen, nutrients, information signaling molecules, hormones, metabolic waste products, and red and white blood cells, can flow as freely to and from their various destinations.

Fascia is often described as one of the body's richest and most important *sensory organs*. It contains at least 250 million nerve endings, many more than are in the skin (~200 million) and eyes (~126 million) (Schleip & Stecco, 2021). Most of the body's nerves, which transmit information in the form of electrochemical signals to and from the brain, are embedded in fascia. Because of this, fascia is an important part of the body's multifaceted *information communication system* that generates, spreads, and responds to chemical, physical, electrical, magnetic, and emotional information between the body's cells, tissues, organs and organ systems. Fascia accordingly plays a significant role in the coordination of all of the body's activities, and its experiencing of pain.

Table 5.4
Functions of fascia

This table highlights some of fascia's better-known functions. There are several recognised others, and probably quite a few more that are still waiting to be discovered.

Fascia is an indispensable member of the body's immune defence system. Some of its many tasks include, but are by no means limited to: supporting the integrity of the skin to help prevent the entry of harmful micro-organisms and chemicals; insulating the body against heat and cold; allowing the body's many parts to move without harmfully rubbing or being torn; preventing the same parts from being compressed and stretched too far apart; absorbing shock; containing and limiting the spread of extravascular (escaped) blood, infection and tumours; providing the space and resources required for the body's immune defense battles; and storing surplus energy as fat, so it is available in times of need.

"The fascial system surrounds, infuses with, and has the potential to influence profoundly every muscle, bone, nerve, blood vessel, organ, and cell of the body. Fascia also separates, supports, connects, and protects everything. This three-dimensional web of connective tissue is alive and ever changing as the body demands. Thus it is a network for information exchange, influencing and influenced by every structure, system, and cell in the organism. Like air and gravity, its influence is so all-pervasive that we have tended to take it for granted." *(Barnes, 1990, pp. xi & 3)*

"Fascia is a cacophony of functions and information … The fascial system supports, protects, evolves and connects the human body." *(Bordoni & Simonelli, 2018)*

The Living Wetsuit

Wetsuits

In my younger 'confront the fear by doing it anyway' days, I learned to scuba dive – to swim below the ocean's surface with a tank of pressurised air strapped on my back. This opened the door to a myriad of magnificent experiences – like the jokey yet life-savingly-serious camaraderie with one's diving buddies, swirling forests of brightly coloured seaweed, a column of fish slowly revolving around a shaft of sunlight, parrot fish encased in their mucous sleeping bubbles, the sinuous flow of a passing sea snake, joining (from a safe distance) the tidal flight of a cluster of giant eagle rays and bronze whaler sharks over a Balinese reef, etc., etc., etc.

Our bodies are designed so they can be safely immersed, move around, and swim within water – provided we don't stray out of our depth, or stay in it for too long. Staying alive when scuba diving ultimately depends on our continuing to breathe air, keeping our bodies sufficiently warm, and maybe not getting attacked by something that fancies us for dinner. The breathing air part is fairly straightforward when we're close to the surface. If we stray too far from our above-water air supply, we need to use some special underwater breathing equipment. Either that,

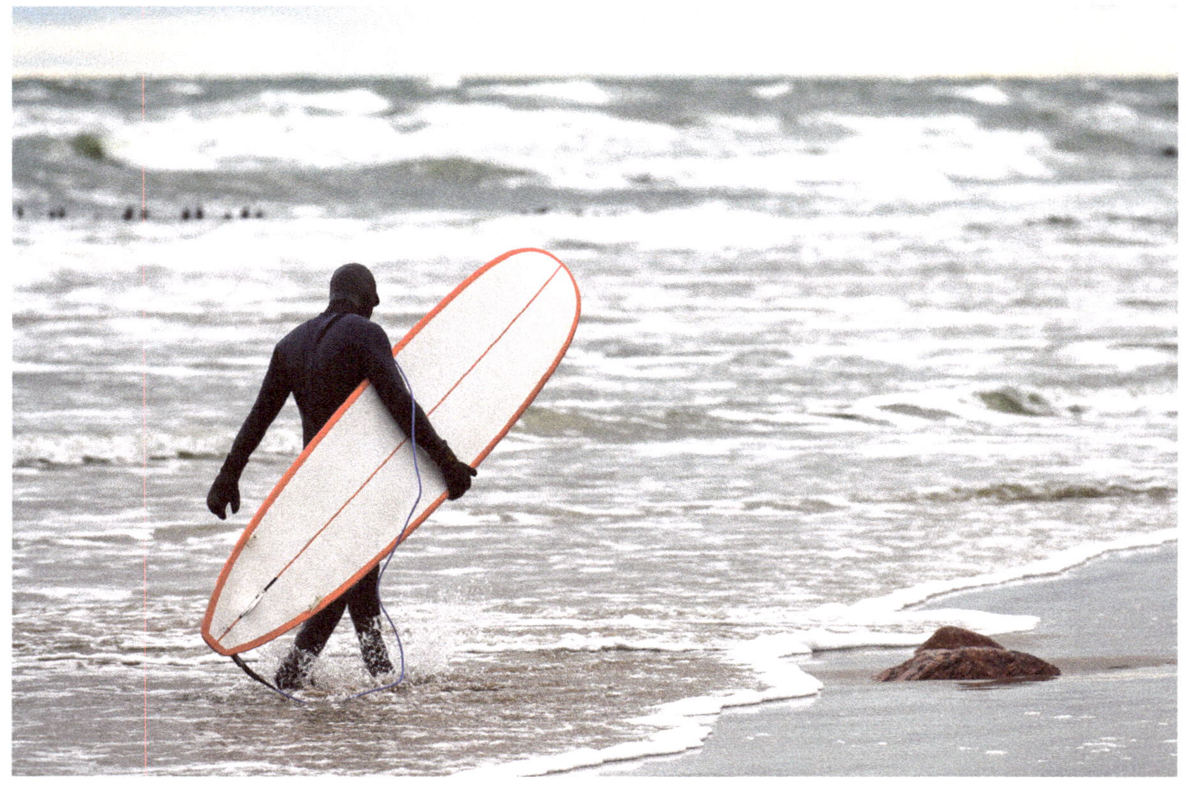

or be extraordinarily skilled at holding our breath – which some people (but not me) are.

Water is a highly efficient conductor of heat – at least 20 times more so than still air. This means that our bodies rapidly get cold when submerged in water that is cooler than them. That is, unless we actively do something to prevent this ... like wearing a wetsuit (see Figure 6.1). There's not all that much we can do about the dinner-menu side of things apart from avoiding attracting unwanted attention to ourselves when in shark territory.

A wetsuit is a waterproof form-fitting garment that covers the outside of a person's body right next to their skin. Wearing a wetsuit helps prevent their body from becoming dangerously chilled (and possibly dying from hypothermia) when they are immersed in, or sprayed by, cold water for a prolonged period of time. It also helps protect them from being physically injured by, for example, sharp objects, coral grazes, and jellyfish stings. Wetsuits are therefore worn by many groups of people, including: recreational, military, and industrial underwater divers; commercial and spear fishermen; sea rescue personnel; surfers, windsurfers, and other sports enthusiasts (e.g., canoeists, cavers, ocean swimmers, and sailors).

Wetsuits are named for the small amount of water that is trapped in a thin layer between their fabric and their wearer's skin. Despite their snug fit, a small amount of cold water from the outside manages to seep in through the wetsuit's neck, wrist, and ankle openings when their wearer first enters the water. Once it has gotten in, this thin layer of trapped water is soon warmed by the wearer's body heat. The warm water, and the body it covers, are then both kept warm by the wetsuit that covers them.

Most of a wetsuit's heat retention capacity comes from its specially designed fabric. Wetsuits are usually made out of foamed neoprene, a sponge-rubber-like material that contains lots of tiny bubbles of nitrogen gas. Nitrogen is a poor thermal conductor (compared to water), which means it doesn't easily conduct heat. The small nitrogen bubbles in the wetsuit fabric lessen the transference of heat from the person wearing the wetsuit into the water that surrounds them, extending the time they can safely stay in a wet and cold environment.

Each garment is assembled by gluing, sewing, and taping together several specially-shaped cut-out-pieces of neoprene sheeting. There are quite a few different types of wetsuits, all of which correspond to a particular set of end-use-relating design specifications. Some are mass-produced in standard adult and child sizes, while others are personalised to fit a customer's body. A 'full length suit' protects most of the body between the base of the neck, ankles and wrists. A 'shorty' usually ends just above the elbows and knees. And a 'long-john' (which has no sleeves but reaches the ankle) is often worn underneath a separate, torso-covering jacket. These garments seldom extend over the wearer's head, hands and feet, so are often worn in conjunction with accessories that cover, insulate, and protect these parts of the body – such as thin-soled neoprene boots and gloves, and a head-covering hood.

A living fleshy human garment

Now, let's see if you can imagine a very different type of 'wetsuit' – a *living, fleshy, skeleton-hugging body garment.* This type of 'wetsuit' is biologically-made and is worn by *every single person* who is (and ever was) alive on this planet. It organically supports and enables everything its human wearer is and does throughout their mortal lifetime.

This soft, human body-shaped garment is worn *underneath* instead of *over* the skin (see Figure 6.2). It surrounds the body's skeleton of bones, and fills up all of the space between them and the body's outer skin surface. This 'living wetsuit's' warm and moist fabric contains and protects all of the body's soft inside 'parts' – including its heart and lungs, its nerves and blood vessels, its muscles and brain. It connects them all together, uniting them into a whole body and prevents them all from collapsing into an icky heap on the ground. When it is alive, this whole-body garment is infused with and exudes several types of energy.[19] These energies of life stop and disappear when the person wearing it dies – which means they cannot be discerned by anatomists working with embalmed cadavers.

Even though this may well be the first time you've tried to conjure up such an image, the notion of a human skeleton clad in fleshy clothing is far from new. People have long known that their physical bodies have soft and hard bits inside them – i.e., their flesh and bones. In animals, including humans, the word *flesh* relates to all of the softish and potentially edible juicy-fatty-meaty

19 Some of the different forms of energy associated with living human bodies include chemical energy, *ch'i*, elastic potential energy, electrical energy, electromagnetic force fields, kinetic energy (energy of motion), non-classical force fields, photonic energy (light), *prana*, sound energy, thermal energy (heat), and quantum fields.

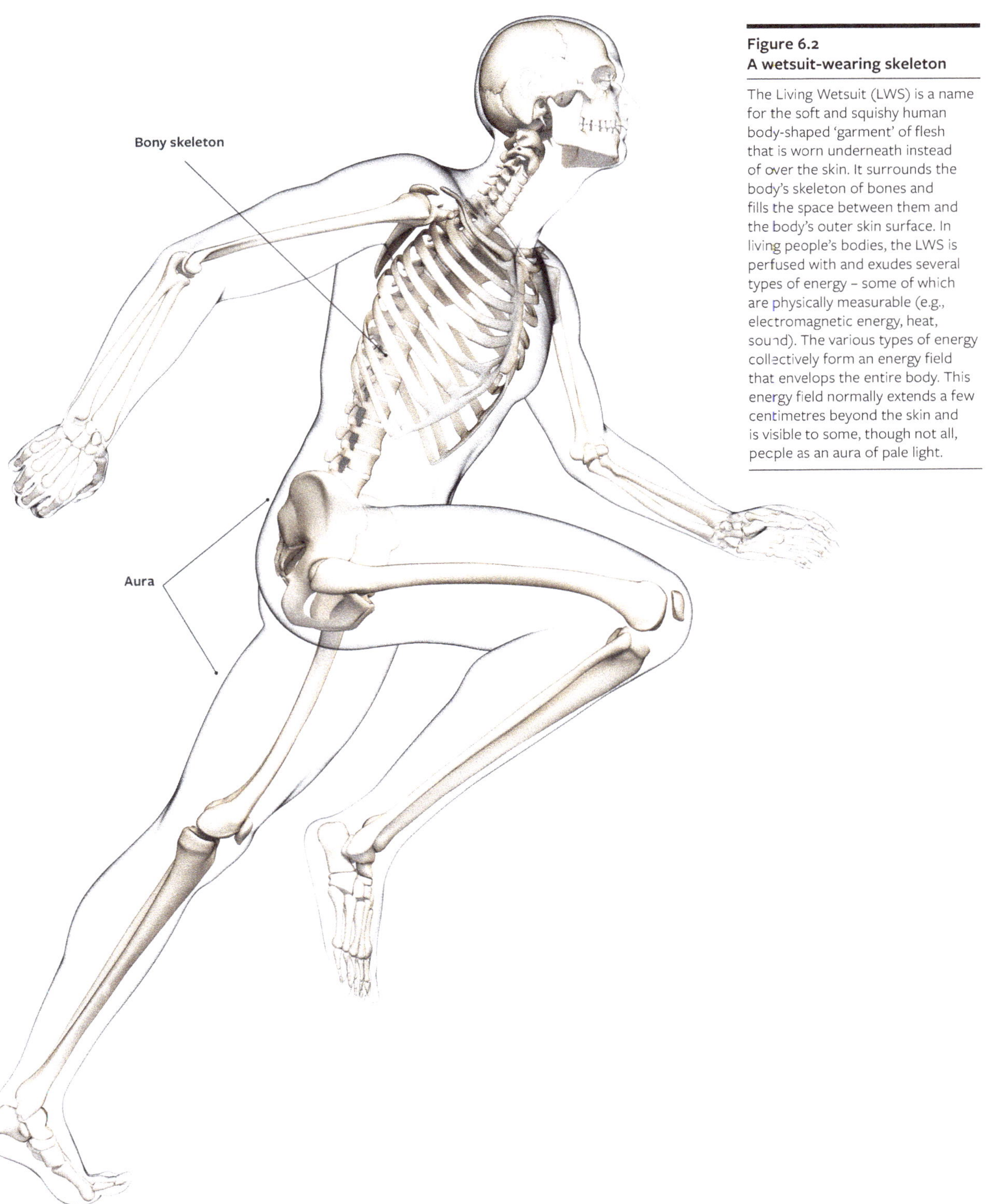

Figure 6.2
A wetsuit-wearing skeleton

The Living Wetsuit (LWS) is a name for the soft and squishy human body-shaped 'garment' of flesh that is worn underneath instead of over the skin. It surrounds the body's skeleton of bones and fills the space between them and the body's outer skin surface. In living people's bodies, the LWS is perfused with and exudes several types of energy – some of which are physically measurable (e.g., electromagnetic energy, heat, sound). The various types of energy collectively form an energy field that envelops the entire body. This energy field normally extends a few centimetres beyond the skin and is visible to some, though not all, people as an aura of pale light.

stuff that covers and envelops their bones. Flesh is vitally important when an animal or person is alive, as it normally provides most of the body's physical bulk, and is in many ways involved in all of the body's activities and processes of living – e.g., walking, breathing, immune defence, and digestion. Without going too far into any of the many-possible gory details, most people also know that the body's covering of flesh (its fleshy garment) decomposes and disintegrates fairly soon after death – especially in hot climates, or if hungry predators have been involved.

The bones, in comparison, are more durable. Most can remain largely intact, as lifeless versions of their former selves, for many years, centuries, and even millennia after their fleshy clothing has disappeared. Because of its relative durability, the skeleton – the body's internal bony framework – is at times analogously equated with the body itself (see Figure 6.3). This is seen, for example, in several old Anglo-Saxon terms for the human body – *ban-hus* ('bone house'), *bansele* ('bone hall'), *ban-fæt* ('bone vessel'), *ban-cofa* ('bone dwelling'), and *ban-loca* ('bone enclosure'). The body's living inhabitant, its soul's enlivening spirit, was in turn known as a ban-huses weard ('the bone house's ward', or protective guardian) (Crystal, 2011).

Since time immemorial, many people have accepted that their bodies consist of more than just flesh and bones. They have realised that people's bodies are not the same as their corpses. Their living bodies seem to contain something else, an animating spirit that somehow goes away and is absent after they have died. We may not be able to physically see or touch this life-giving energy force, it is generally not mentioned in today's anatomy and medical textbooks, yet its presence has been extensively acknowledged in many different parts of the world for eons.[20] Without it, the body is dead – whether or not we explicitly acknowledge its existence, or even give it a name.

A person's soul, according to this overall way of thinking about things, is the putative source of the vitalising life energy

20　Even though the soul and its body-enlivening life force are widely recognised as an integral part of a person's living body, they are normally overlooked by today's Western world anatomists. This is understandable, as they can only describe the things they can scientifically see and photograph, touch, count and measure. The soul and its associated range of subtle energy phenomena generally do not fall into this category. They are normally long gone by the time the body's physical remnants turn up in the anatomy lab. Yet, it is important to remember that *an absence of scientific evidence is not the same as evidence of absence*. Several of the body's non-physical vitalising energy structures are, and have long been, apparent to suitably skilled observers (including Yeshi Dhonden, who was mentioned in Chapter 2). Although they may not be acknowledged in our Western anatomical and medical textbooks, these intangible human body elements are prominently featured in many other cultural groups' spiritual and medical traditions.

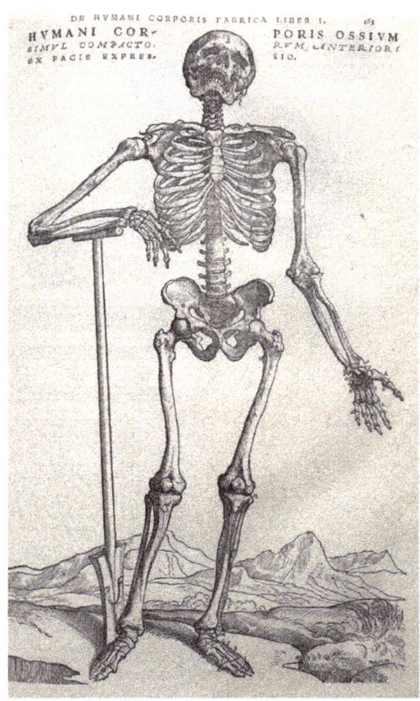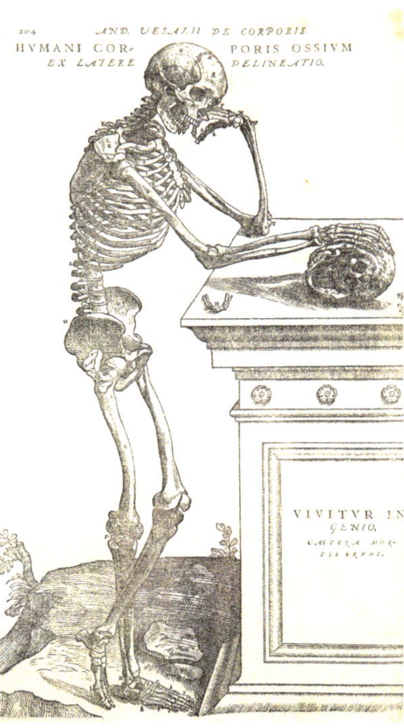

Figure 6.3
Bony people

Artists have long used pictures of skeletons to represent people's bodies. These woodcut illustrations used by Vesalius (1543, pp. 163 & 164), for example, symbolically reduce the body to its bare bones.

force that flows through each person's body during the course of their entire lifetime, imbuing it with their personal mix of moral, intellectual, spiritual, and emotional qualities. The soul is immortal whereas its biological body garment is not. They part company when a person dies. The earthly body is left behind to physically break down, while the soul, so it is said, survives forever in another, timeless state of being.

The life-giving energy that infuses and animates each person's flesh-and-bones body is known by a variety of names in different cultural settings. Some of these include:

- Pneuma (Ancient Greek)
- Ch'i or qi (Chinese)
- Ki (Japanese)
- Prana (Indian)

- Mana (Hawaiian)

- Mauri (New Zealand Maori)

- Élan vital (French)

- Life force or life energy

- Impulse of life

- Astral light

- Vital energy/principle/spark/spirit

- Spiritual essence

- Breath of life

The Living Wetsuit

The Living Wetsuit (LWS) is a simple and easy to understand anatomical analogy that relates to a person's whole and life-energy-infused fleshy body garment. This contemporary conceptual model provides an uncomplicated way of understanding our body's naturally whole and alive, rather than its dead and anatomised, structure. This way of depicting the human body also uniquely incorporates two very important things that have traditionally received relatively little, if any, of the anatomy profession's descriptive attention. These are, (1) the fascia that connects the body's unnaturally separated (dissected) 'parts' together and makes the body whole, and (2) the subtle life-endowing energy force that animates a person's living body. Our bodies would not be what they are and could not work without both of these things, so it is important to acknowledge their existence – even if they may be somewhat tricky to explain.

Of course there are many differences between living and neoprene wetsuits, yet the LWS, as you might expect, is far more complex and interesting than its neoprene counterpart can ever be. Simply put, these living fleshy, skeleton-hugging body garments are:

The Living Wetsuit is an anatomical analogy for a person's whole and life-energy-infused fleshy body garment.

64

- *Designed and made by Mother Nature* rather than by people, computers, and machines. LWSs are mind-bogglingly complex and contain a wide variety of components, all of which are seamlessly fitted together. Each LWS is similar but different to everyone else's. It is uniquely configured to the needs of its owner. These high-performance human garments are made of a natural, living biological material – i.e., warm and moist human tissue, rather than rubbery factory-made stuff. A LWS generates and regulates its own heat levels (through a mix of metabolic, movement, and insulation mechanisms) and, when needs be, can be boosted by the wearing of clothes – including neoprene wetsuits.

- *Naturally whole.* A LWS comes in one whole-body-shaped unit that includes its head, face, hands and feet rather than several pieces that have been joined together. LWSs are, in general, aesthetically pleasant to look at. Each has an inbuilt shape memory, so it can resume its normal shape and properties after being (moderately) stretched or compressed. They are normally flexible and comfortable to wear – so much so that it is easy for its wearer to forget that they are wearing it.

- *Normally strong and resilient.* LWSs are physically tough and flexible at the same time. They are durable and puncture resistant, and are resistant to tearing. They absorb and transmit strain, and provide impact protection during normal use and minor collisions or falls. They tolerate heating and cooling, and protect the body against a variety of potentially lethal hazards. They are waterproof and watertight – i.e., they remain intact when immersed in water and don't have any potentially leaky seams.

- *Sensitive, sentient and smart.* A LWS houses the body's nervous system – i.e., the brain and spinal cord and the network of autonomic, motor and sensory nerves and nerve endings that connects to them.[21] In effect, this means that the LWS can sense and respond to all sorts of things that are (or maybe are not) continuously happening inside and near to it. This ability to feel and respond is essential in maintaining a relatively stable and life-sustaining equilibrium (homeostatic balance) between all of its interdependent structural and functional parts and processes. In this way, the LWS is sensitive, perceptive, and communicative. It is also sentient and smart – i.e., it is conscious and appropriately responsive to most of the things that are happening in and to it.

- *Adaptive.* No two LWSs are exactly the same because each LWS adapts to accommodate and safely support its wearer's particular and ever-changing set of bio-chemical, biomechanical, cultural, emotional, energetic, environmental, health, intellectual, psychical, physical, and physiological conditions and requirements. This means that LWSs can adjust their size and shape to match, for example, their wearer's age and life stage development and growth, lifestyle and body-use, injuries and or physical fitness levels.

- *Vibrant and alive.* The LWS hosts and dynamically participates in the integrated activity of all of its wearer's organ systems (e.g., cardiovascular, digestive, endocrine, immune, musculoskeletal, respiratory). It is electrically active, conductive, and responsive. It contains lots of fluid, and helps regulate and balance the streams of fluid and energy that flow through it, carrying their respective cargoes of nutrients and waste products, information and migrant cells, oxygen and carbon dioxide. As long as

21 Including those that surround the nerves, blood and lymphatic vessels inside the body's bones.

it is alive, the LWS is constantly in motion. Its molecules vibrate. Its cells change their shape. Its organs pulse with their own rhythms, and move in relation to each other. Its muscles contract, often causing the body's limbs to move and possibly change their positioning.

- *Worn by everyone for all of their lives*, not just those whose bodies need to be protected while they are temporarily in a cold and watery environment. LWSs are energy efficient and reliable. They are also easy to clean – which is good as they are worn all of the time. A LWS is consistently protective and supportive of its wearer. Even when it becomes a bit tired and timeworn, this special garment somehow or other copes with all of life's stages, conditions and challenges, until it can't and it (and its wearer) dies. After that, it quietly disintegrates and (if let to its own devices) organically disappears in an environmentally responsible manner.

In my many years of clinical and teaching experience, I've observed that the LWS anatomy model's practical and down-to-earth logic instantly makes sense to most people – not just those with university degrees, white lab coats, or medical jobs. I've continually seen people from 8–93 years of age 'get it' and 'use it' in less than a minute, and then continue to use it at home *because it makes sense and works for them.*

Some of them have later told me that they've liked this no-nonsense way of understanding their body so much, and have found it so useful in helping them care for their bodies, that they've passed it on to their family and friends – who've promptly latched onto it too. That has potential to advance the ways we understand how our bodies work and may be more comprehensively cared for.

The Body's Fabric of Life

07

"Connectivity and unity are organismic truths."
(Agneessens, 2001, p. 22)

Living Wetsuit fabric

The Living Wetsuit (LWS), a person's whole and life-energy-infused fleshy body garment, is made from a special type of biological fabric. This living textile surrounds, interweaves between, and infiltrates everything else in the body – including its organs and skeleton of bones. Its soft three-dimensional web of tissue connects all of the body's so-called parts, uniting them into a single body whole. No wonder it – i.e., fascia – has been called the body's *fabric of wholeness* (Agneessens, 2001). Our bodies simply could not exist without it.

Our bodies' web of fascial fabric is like a living, three-dimensional version of a cotton needlepoint canvas. A completed piece of needlepoint – the sort of thing that might, for instance, cover a cushion – is created by embellishing its canvas with a mass of colourful embroidery stitches (see Figure 7.1). Each tiny stitch is formed when the embroiderer inserts a short length of dyed cotton, silk, or wool needlepoint yarn into its designated place within the canvas's lattice of threads. The multi-hued pattern of stitches is primarily responsible for the needlepoint's eventual decorative appearance.

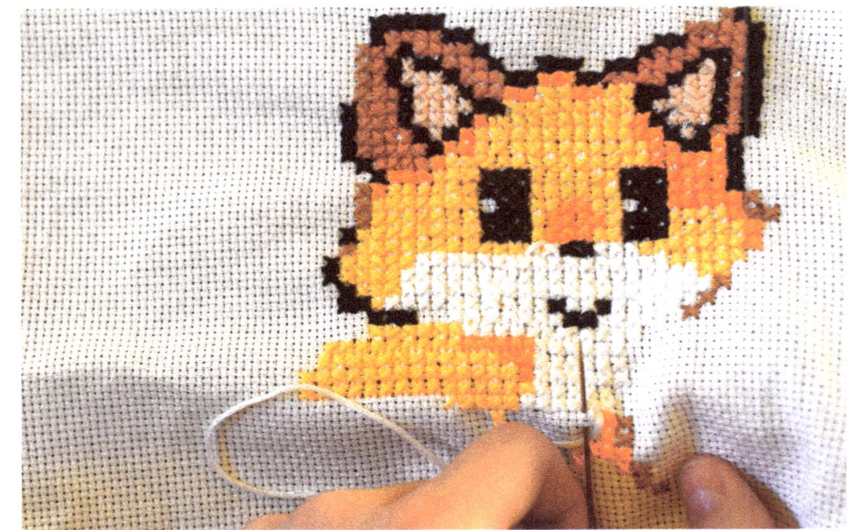

A person's LWS fabric is obviously not the same as a finished piece of needlepoint. It is considerably more complex (on all sorts of levels) than its inanimate counterpart. In spite of this, both are made of a relatively inconspicuous mesh material that has lots of colourful and eye-catching things embedded in it. A work of needlepoint starts with a piece of whitey-beigey canvas that is subsequently obscured from view by the embroiderer's stitches. The LWS fabric is instead a person-shaped web of pale fascial tissue that has lots of interesting biological bits and pieces set in it – including muscle cells, nerves, blood vessels, Type I collagen fibres, and bones.

Cotton needlepoint canvas and the body's fascial fabric may each be described in their own right. As can the yarn and 'biological stitches' inserted into them. Both of these things – the basic material and the multi-coloured things set in it – are required to create the finished result. The end product, however, is not the same as the components that went into its making. It is something altogether new and different.

"[T]he whole is something else than the sum of the parts"
(Koffka, 1935, p. 176)

Parenchyma and stroma

Nowadays, the words *parenchyma* and *stroma* are used to distinguish the two main elements that make up a body organ, such as a liver or a muscle. Parenchyma refers to the groups of cells that perform that organ's special functional tasks. Fascia, the seemingly nondescript tissue that encases, connects, and supports the organ's parenchymal parts, equates to its stroma (see Figure 7.2).

The parenchyma of liver, for example, contains lots of liver cells (*hepatocytes*) whose job includes cleaning the blood and making proteins. A muscle similarly contains lots of muscle cells. When they get excited, they contract and tighten. They get shorter and fatter, pushing and pulling into the fascial stroma that surrounds them, often causing something near them to move – such as a blood vessel, or maybe a bone.

This is the point where many people's understandings of livers and muscles pretty much begins and ends. As far as they are concerned, livers are made of liver cells, and muscles are made of muscle cells. While there is *some* truth in both of these assumptions, neither are fully true. Livers *contain* lots of liver cells, and muscles *contain* lots of muscle cells … all of which are implanted in the organ's ubiquitous stroma, its fascial canvas. Knowing about the parenchymal cells is really useful, because it helps us understand *some* of what these organs do. But not all. Our knowledge of what they do, and how they do it, will inevitably be limited unless we also take the stroma's contribution into account.

Anatomists and other scientists have regularly paid considerably more attention to examining the body's parenchymal bits than their stromal counterparts. Most of their interest has been directed towards the things they can easily see and have thought to be more functionally important – such as muscle cells and liver cells. The less obvious and relatively less interesting to look at fascial stroma, on the other hand, hasn't attracted nearly as much of their attention. French anatomist and pathologist

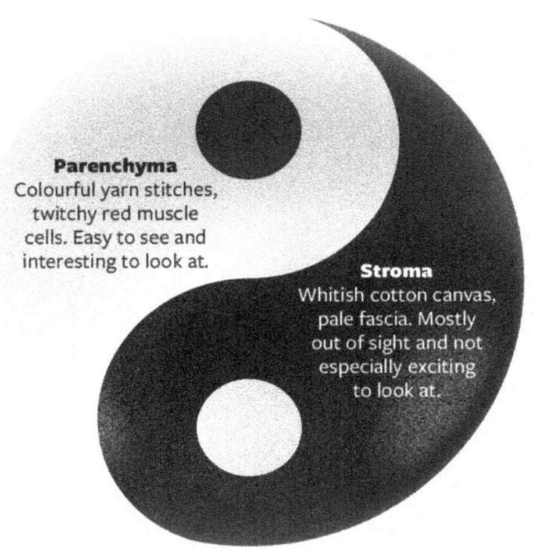

Figure 7.2
Parenchyma and stroma

The ancient Chinese yin and yang symbol is used here to demonstrate the coming together of two different things to create a new something-else. Separately, each thing (e.g., parenchyma and stroma) has its own identity and qualities. Then, when they are united, they become something else. Both things are equally as essential in the making of the new whole, even if one may at first seem more important than the other. The new whatever-it-is could not exist without the union of both components.

Xavier Bichat (1771–1802) acknowledged this rarely mentioned oversight. In his words, fascia (which he then called membranes) has not

> … hitherto been a particular object of research among anatomists. This kind of organs (sic), disseminated as it were (sic) through all the others, contributing to the structure of most of them, and having rarely a separate existence, have never been separately examined by them. Their history has been associated with that of the organs over which they are spread. The pericardium and the heart, the pleura and the lungs [etc.] … For description, this is doubtless the best and most simple progress; but in following it, anatomists, struck with the different structure of the organs, have forgotten that their respective membranes could possess any analogy; they have neglected to establish any relation between them, and this leaves an essential chasm. (1813, p. 21)

Individual exceptions notwithstanding (e.g., Still, 1899; Gallaudet, 1931; Stilwell, 1957), it took nearly 200 more years before that state of affairs began to significantly change. For most of that period, fascia was simply regarded as an inert kind of tissue that passively invests, contains, separates, covers, obscures and fills the gaps in between all of the other, *higher* (Gallaudet, 1931), or *more specialised* (Jones, 1943), parts of the body, such as muscles and bones and visceral organs. Fascia's natural transparency and general lack of colour when alive made it difficult to see anything but the whitish, Type I collagen-reinforced sections of it during surgery. It was also routinely 'cleaned' away by anatomists who wanted to study the body's more definite other parts. All of this has helped prevent many people from realising that their body's organs – including its muscles and liver, and heart – are not entirely made of parenchymal cells. These organs can neither exist nor work without the fascial stroma that supports their cells. By the same token, the organ's fascial stroma is but a 'ghost' of its normal self without its usual complement of parenchymal cells.[22]

Fascia "sheathes, permeates, divides and subdivides every portion of all animal bodies, surrounding and penetrating every muscle and all its fibers – every artery, and every fiber and principle thereunto belonging, and ... the venous system with its great company of lymphatics ... It belts each muscle, vein, nerve, and all organs of the body ... By its action we live, and by its failure we shrink, or swell, and die." *(Still, 1899, pp. 163–164)*

"Though a practical impossibility, if you could leave the fascia intact and remove everything else from the body (bones, nerves, organs, arteries and veins, etc.) you would be left with a kind of three-dimensional blueprint of the body – in essence, a fascial body. It would look something like a huge loofa sponge in the shape of your body. In it, you could see where every single bone, nerve, blood vessel, organ, and so forth belongs. Reverse the image for a moment. Imagine that you could remove all the fascia from the body. Aside from the bones and a few other structures, what you would see remaining would be a heap of unrecognizable, formless, organic stuff."
(Maitland, 1995, p. 153)

22 This book deliberately does not contain any photographs of human tissue due to their potential to distress some readers. If this is not of concern for you, and you would like to see what a human heart looks like with and without its parenchymal cells, see: https://m.facebook.com/TheFasciaConnection/posts/from-fascia-research-congress-ivchapter-1-fascia-and-anatomydo-you-wonder-how-mu/763084623871355/

Myofascia

The word myofascia began to appear in the mid-20th century medical discussion of the newly identified *myofascial pain syndromes*. Myofascia is a concept that acknowledges the natural juxtaposition of muscle cells (*myo-*) and fascia (*-fascia*) in the organs that anatomists have long known as muscles. Muscle cells are usually red coloured, so it's fairly easy to see them (compared to the largely colourless fascial substance that surrounds them).

To this day, muscles are widely envisaged as a mass of reddish parenchymal cells that contract and induce movement (by pulling lengthwise through the tendons that connect their ends to bone). This understanding is only half-true as it fails to account for the muscles' fascial stroma. Yet, despite this obvious shortcoming in logic, this abbreviated idea anatomically under-pins the *musculoskeletal* approach to body treatment (which has a strong local focus on muscles, tendons, bones, joints, ligaments, and nerves) that is currently provided by a host of health practitioners – including, for example, many physiotherapists, physical and rehabilitation medicine specialists, sports physicians, and orthopaedic surgeons.

On average, about one third of a person's body mass is muscle (Janssen et al., 2000), though not all of that muscle mass is made of parenchymal muscle cells. In reality, fascia surrounds and connects every skeletal muscle fibre, bundles of muscle fibres, muscle, and groups of muscles – endowing each with its special structural form (see Figure 7.3). Fascia makes it possible for all of them to move friction-freely beside each other and the tissue that adjoins them without being damaged. It absorbs the changes in pressure generated by the contracting muscle cells. It disperses the resulting push-and-pull forces three-dimensionally through the muscle's (intramuscular) interior and its exterior (epimuscular) surroundings, including but not only its tendon (Huijing, 2009). Fascia also houses the blood and lymphatic vessels, the nerves and the interstitial fluid flows that nourish a muscle's cells, and then clears away their waste products. It contains most of the body's sensory nerve endings and nerves, hence senses and helps expedite the vital flow of information between the muscle and the rest of its owner's body. Muscles do not exist and cannot work without fascia. This is why they are sometimes, and perhaps more correctly, described as *myofascial body units* (Myers, 2014).

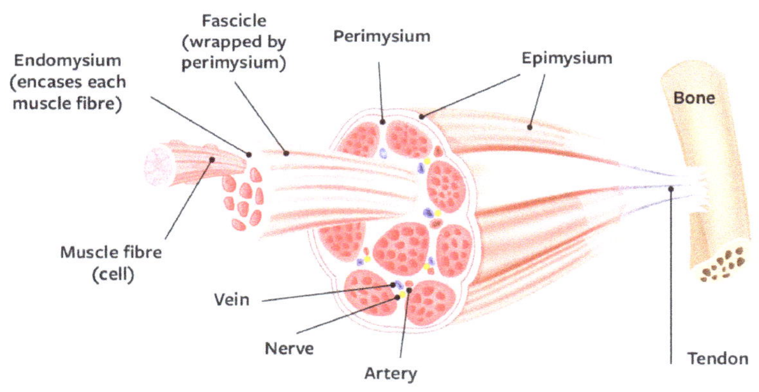

Figure 7.3
Myofascia (muscle + fascia)

A muscle's stroma is generally described in relation to the fascial tissue that is wrapped around three differently sized groups of muscle cells: (1) the *endomysium* that overlies the sarcolemma (muscle cell membrane), which encases each muscle fibre (muscle cell); (2) the *perimysium* that encases each bundle (fascicle) of muscle fibres; and (3) the *epimysium* that encases the muscle. Despite their different names, the endo-, peri- and epi-mysium are continuous with each other and the rest of the body's universal fascial matrix.

"There is no such thing as a muscle … every muscle of the body is surrounded by a smooth fascial sheath, every muscular fascicle is surrounded by fascia, every fibril is surrounded by fascia, and every microfibril down to cellular level is surrounded by fascia. Therefore, it is the fascia that ultimately determines the length and function of its muscular component … [The] separation of the fascia and its influence from the muscular component and their influence on each other is imaginary."
(Barnes, 1990, pp. 3 & 5)

Whole and alive

The LWS's biological fabric physical structure is, as explained earlier in this chapter, somewhat like an elaborate piece of needlepoint. The way the LWS fabric works may instead be compared to a bustling modern city. A quick look at a decent map shows that the entire city is topographically arranged around an extensive network of variously sized motorways, highways, roads, bridges, tunnels, streets, avenues, boulevards, lanes, alleys, tracks, footpaths, driveways, stairways, lift-shafts, corridors, and hallways (cf. the city's stromal canvas). The interconnecting web of thoroughfares is interspersed with a diverse mix of buildings and rooms (cf. the city's parenchymal embroidery stitches) – each of which is in some way capable of contributing to its neighbourhood's, and the city's, special functioning and character. The city's roads and buildings on their own, however, are not enough to make that city function as it was designed to do. To make the city a real city, to make it hum with activity and purpose, it also needs something else. It needs people to energise it and bring it to life. Without them, it is just a soulless city-shell rather than a whole and living city-organism.

Our whole and life infused LWS is in many ways like a city populated by people. It provides our bodies with their soft fleshy structure and dynamically participates in all of their processes of living.

> "Fascia forms an integrating tissue system that unifies
> the body connecting all parts together. It helps all areas
> of the body to work together in coordinated patterns of
> movement. Therefore, the structure and function of each
> individual part of the body as a whole is to some extent
> controlled by the fascia. As a result, fascia has an important
> role in maintaining our health." *(Michael Kern 2001, p. 81)*

When Things Start to Go Wrong with the Living Wetsuit

Kahu's story

I was recently asked to make a home-visit to see 'Kahu',[23] a friend-of-a-friend who'd been stuck in bed for nearly a month with an extremely bad headache. The pain relief and anti-anxiety medication prescribed by Kahu's regular doctor hadn't even slightly helped lessen his problem, so he'd been admitted to hospital for some more specialised medical attention. Thankfully, the relevant barrage of hospital tests showed he didn't have a dangerous life-threatening condition, like a brain haemorrhage or brain cancer. Yet, the doctors also couldn't find anything anywhere else in his body, or mind, that could be causing such serious head pain. Their hands were tied without a firm diagnosis, so Kahu was eventually discharged home the following week, with several new packets of hospital-strength pills ... *and* his horrible headache.

When I saw Kahu several days later, he was still bedridden, still in a lot of pain, and he couldn't move his head the tiniest bit without feeling sick. He was also, by now, getting really worried about his future. What *was* causing his headache? Was there

23   This story about 'Kahu' is based on my experience of treating several people with similar health issues in different parts of New Zealand. The different happenings in this case narrative are all real, in that they all truly happened. I have blended them together into one composite story, in order to protect the anonymity of the individuals concerned, and to illustrate their shared experiences more compellingly.

something seriously wrong with his body? How much longer would he be so unwell? What would happen if he didn't get better?

I sat down on the edge of his bed, and carefully listened to his account of what was going on. To the distress being voiced in his painfully murmured narrative. His desperation to recover and begin living again. I noticed the ways he held his body and avoided moving it unless he absolutely had to. The ways he did and didn't breathe. The raised tight lumps and cords of muscle in his neck and shoulders. His dull eyes, and stale invalid's breath. His pallid and dehydrated skin. He certainly was not imagining his pain. Something *was* definitely wrong, and hopefully it could soon be found and treated.

To cut a long story short, everything I heard and saw indicated to me that Kahu's LWS might contain some problematic tight spots that were, in effect, causing it to shrink and twist. If so, it was possible that some headache-inducing body parts in his head-neck-shoulder area (i.e., nerves, blood vessels, joints between bones, and fasciae) were being abnormally stretched or compressed, and, in turn, had become sore and inflamed.

With his permission, I put my hands on his skin and gently eased a few of the most obvious tight spots in his shoulders and neck. Ten minutes later, Kahu's headache was easing, and, after another few minutes of treatment, it had stopped – for the first time since it began! He breathed a deep sigh of relief, and his body visibly relaxed. His eyes and skin had brightened. His voice sounded more real. He test-rolled his head from side-to-side, and then smiled.

Kahu had easily understood my explanations about why and what I was doing during his treatment. The idea of his body being like a LWS-wearing skeleton made perfect sense to him. Loosening up the tight spots in its fabric seemed pretty logical, especially as he had just felt what happened when this was done. He was feeling much better in himself and had reason to hope that his health might continue to improve. His life might (fingers crossed) bearably begin again.

I told Kahu that it was unlikely that this one brief treatment would completely and permanently solve his headache problem. It was an encouraging start, especially as we had discovered that something *could* be done to help relieve his pain. Now he needed to learn a few things *he* could do to help progress his recovery, after I left his hometown later that day. Kahu welcomed the idea of helping himself heal (in tandem with his doctors' advice) – by doing things such as keeping his body well hydrated and warm. Remembering to breathe into the whole, rather than just at the top, of his lungs. Gently moving and stretching all of his body while he was lying in bed, with his head and neck comfortably supported by pillows. Going for short walks inside the house, and later his garden, when he felt well enough to do so. Then, if and when it felt right, to consider finding a nearby fascia-aware bodywork practitioner who could help him improve the way his LWS fitted his body's skeleton, as a whole.

I'm not a hot-shot-miracle-healer, so what happened? Why could I see something (which was really obvious to me) that the doctors hadn't? I think my being able to help Kahu boiled down to the fact that my understanding of the body includes fascia. This meant I knew about and *could be* interested in the condition of his LWS … and was then able to see if it might have something to do with his headache. This way of thinking about the body's structure (and headaches) is not going to help everyone all of the time. Then again, it can be really useful to have it up our sleeve, especially when facing a mystifying and (seemingly) tricky-to-solve health problem.

Tight spots

Unfortunately, a LWS is not always in its best or most healthy condition. Life happens, though not always in ways we would choose. LWSs are worn all of the time – 24/7 all the way through their wearers' lives. They are sometimes born with a few structural or functional problems (e.g., an interventricular septal heart defect), and are highly likely to develop several more over the years. They are constantly working and moving, and continue to do so in all sorts of conditions. They are resilient and normally long-living, yet most of them eventually experience a few injuries and health problems. Our LWSs can easily become a bit too tight or sore in places. In others they may be overstretched or twisted out of shape. If doctors think the problems are medically serious enough they are usually given medical names, such as arthritis, chronic back pain, Dupuytren's contracture, myofascial pain syndrome, plantar-fasciitis, and tennis elbow.

Over time, nearly everyone's LWS develops a number of *tight spots* – variously-sized places where the LWS's fabric has become thicker than normal, less pliable, and tender to touch. They may be hot or painful, though they often aren't. And, even if they are, they don't show up on plain X-rays, which means their symptom-causing presence more often than not remains unnoticed by doctors and other health professionals. Ignoring them could be a mistake, as they can, and frequently do, adversely affect a person's wellbeing and health.

Some types of tight spots are called *trigger points*, others are known as *fascial adhesions*, or *myofascial restrictions*. Others have no special name, they just are places where the LWS fabric is noticeably denser, tenser, and more tender than usual. Tight spots can develop pretty much anywhere in a person's LWS – from the scalp on their head to the soles of their feet, from their skin through to their organs and bones. They commonly crop up in areas where the LWS's fabric has been injured, chronically strained, or maybe not moved enough. They may occur in conjunction with infections, swellings, and scars, or, sometimes, even after a medical injection or a too-vigorous exercise regime. They may also appear in places where nothing untoward seems to have happened, and, at first glance, everything seems perfectly normal (even though it actually isn't).

Tight spots in the LWS can be caused by many things, some of which include:

- Physical trauma
- Overuse injuries
- Lack of exercise/insufficient everyday movement
- Poor posture
- Ill-chosen footwear
- Prolonged immobilisation, splintage, or bedrest
- Chronic pain
- Infection
- Inflammation and swelling
- Surgery
- Acute and chronic medical conditions
- Tattooing
- Irritating chemicals (e.g., insect stings, injections, betel nut juice)
- Hereditary and acquired connective tissue disorders
- Emotional stress
- Tumours
- Radiation and other deep burns
- Dehydration and inadequate nutrition

One thing that tight spots have in common is the way they begin. They all develop in areas of tissue that have for one reason or another become inflamed. Inflammation is LWS's natural defensive response to irritation, injury, and infection. At first, inflammation helps prevent whatever it is that's doing the damage from spreading any further and doing more harm. Next, it cleans up the mess (e.g., cellular debris, microbes, and other contaminants) so that the affected tissue is made ready to be repaired and healed.

The processes of inflammation, tissue repair, healing, and recovery mostly happen in the LWS's fascial ground substance. This ubiquitous gel houses most of the LWS's sentry and signalling cells; immune soldier cells and their chemical weapons; the clean-up-squad and repair-engineer cells; nerves and their neurochemical emissaries; and the fluids and fluid transporting vessels that deliver the necessary supplies, pass on information, and take away the trash. It provides the interstitial (between-cell) battle space, and flexibly expands to temporarily accommodate atypical volumes of cells, blood, inflammatory exudate, pus and other debris. Fascia is the place where the granulation tissue and scar-forming cells work their reparative magic, support the regrowth of that area's specialty-function cells (e.g., muscle cells, liver cells), and thus enable the subsequent revival of its tissues.

Once the first (or acute) stage of inflammation has passed (usually anywhere between a few minutes and a few days) the LWS fabric may or may not return to its normal condition. It often does. But at times it may not, and is left with some residual tight spots – places where fascia's gel substance has become drier and thicker than usual. This in turn reduces the distance between the Type I collagen fibres that are enmeshed in it, making the LWS fabric denser and less pliable. If the space between these fibres decreases and drops below a certain level, they are at risk of becoming electrochemically stuck to each other, as well as to the tissue beside them. The end result is rather like a pile of left-over, cold, cooked spaghetti whose tangled strands have gotten too close, become firmly stuck to each other, and formed a congealed lump.

Inflammation in the LWS

An acute inflammatory response begins within minutes to hours of an area of LWS fabric being sufficiently irritated, stressed or injured (e.g., overstretched, cut, torn, hit, squashed, burned, infected, poisoned, or diseased). The damaged tissue triggers an influx of white blood cells (histiocytes, mast cells). These cells release a surge of inflammation activating chemicals (including cytokines, histamine, kinins, and prostaglandins) that alert the immune defence system to the danger that exists in their territory. Nearby arterioles expand and become more open, allowing an increased flow of blood and heat into the area. The capillary walls become more leaky, enabling inflammatory exudate – a fluid that transports a squad of useful cells (e.g., neutrophils, eosinophils, basophils, and macrophages), proteins (e.g., plasma proteins, antibodies, fibrin, platelets), oxygen, and nutrients – to seep out into the combat zone. Macrophages find and destroy harmful microorganisms and waste and release a crew of cytokine signalling molecules. The blood thickens and forms a clot that seals off any breached blood vessels, thus preventing the escape of too much blood, and also helps block the spread of infection to nearby tissues.

By now, the injured area tissue is usually ready for repair and healing. An ingrowth of tiny capillaries transforms the clot into blood-rich granulation tissue. Fascial fibroblasts and myofibroblasts multiply and bridge the granulation tissue-filled gap with strings of newly secreted collagen fibres. Macrophages continue to remove whatever debris needs clearing, and newly grown epithelial cells cover over the wound surface. The granulation tissue firms up with the incursion of freshly grown collagen and is converted into scar tissue. Myofibroblasts contact and pull on the collagenous fibres, further closing the wound, and, over time, strengthening the scar.

Once the scar has formed and stabilised, the cells that normally function in that area of tissue – e.g., muscle cells, liver cells, nerve cells – begin to regenerate (as much as they are able to). As healing progresses, the tissue gets stronger and better organised, so that it can deal with its own particular workload. This healing stage of recovery can last for many months, even years.

An acute inflammation cycle is short-lived, normally lasting between a few hours and a few days – just long enough for this essential survival mechanism to protect the body from being harmed further, and to repair the damaged tissue. The key signs of acute inflammation are redness, heat, swelling, loss of function (e.g., movement, breathing, sensing touch), and pain.

Chronic inflammation is when the acute inflammatory response fails to eliminate the problem, or just fails to stop. The immune system keeps on trying to get rid of 'the problem,' which may or may not actually exist by then. The inflammation can linger over months-to-years, and the immune cells may broaden their attack to include healthy tissues and organs. In this way, chronic inflammation can become a problem by itself, and plays a central role in several disease conditions (e.g., rheumatoid arthritis, diabetes, asthma, and Alzheimer's disease).

Why tight spots matter

Tight spots are important, and much more so than many people (including lots of health professionals and health insurance companies) may realise. These localised areas of tightening in the LWS can be the source of a considerable amount of discomfort and misery – whether or not we are aware of their existence. Dense and swollen tight spots take up space, so can painfully stretch or squash the things beside them. The pain may vary in intensity, from a mild ache to seriously sore. The pain may come and go or be there all the time. It may also be felt anywhere in the body, close to and even far away from its source.

Tight spots are places where the LWS's fascial substance has become abnormally dehydrated and gummy. It is effectively turned into a glue that sticks things together. This can cause the

Type I collagen fibres, blood and lymphatic vessels, nerves and nerve endings that are set within it to become squished together in a throbbing jumbled lump. The gluey fascial substance may also painfully disrupt the friction-free gliding motion that normally occurs between the things that are embedded within and next to it (e.g., nerves, tendons, bursae). This can interfere with the ability of these things to move independently alongside each other without rubbing and may eventually contribute to the development of local and widespread movement restrictions.

The LWS is whole – it comes in one piece. In this way, everything within it is connected to everything else, wherever they may be physically situated in the body. As its fascial fabric dries and densifies, it shrinks and stiffens so that the LWS as a whole gradually becomes tighter, less flexible and less comfortable to wear. The LWS's innate interconnectedness also means that a tight spot (a localised area of tissue stuckness) can pull and drag into other areas of its fabric – just like when you grip and then pull on a piece of clothing (see Figure 8.1). As time goes by, these pull-strain lines can produce problems far removed from the original area of stuckness. A tight spot at the knee may, for instance, pull up through the thigh into the pelvis, shift the spine and ribcage out of their normal alignment, and strain a shoulder or the neck. The areas of tissue it pulls into (e.g., in the thigh, pelvis, back and neck) may themselves become overstretched, stressed and inflamed, and then develop some new tight spots of their own. In this way, each tight spot has potential to generate its own radiating clusters of pull-strain lines and tight spots.

Between them, tight spots and pull-strain lines can pull and twist the LWS, along with the things – i.e., cells, tissues, organs, organs systems – contained within it. Unless remedied, this is likely to adversely affect the shape, position, relative alignment, functioning, and health of the LWS and its contained 'parts.'

Dense and tense LWS fabric, for example, has less elasticity or 'give,' so is less able to absorb and disperse shock than it normally

Figure 8.1
Effect of tight spots

Tight spots pull on the fleshy fabric around them, much like a snag pulls into a knitted piece of clothing. The pull force may be transmitted through the LWS fabric, via pull-strain lines, and cause some problems (including, for example, inflammation, pain, limitation of movement, and swelling) that are far removed from the site of the original tight spot. This may, for example, cause the LWS to fit tightly over the bones and joints beneath it, or cause the LWS to become twisted or otherwise distorted.

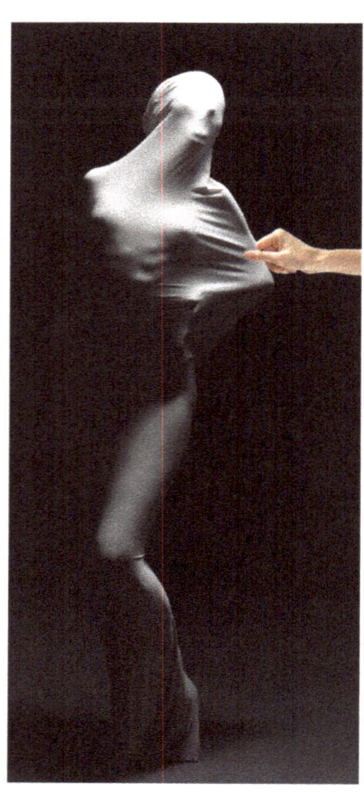

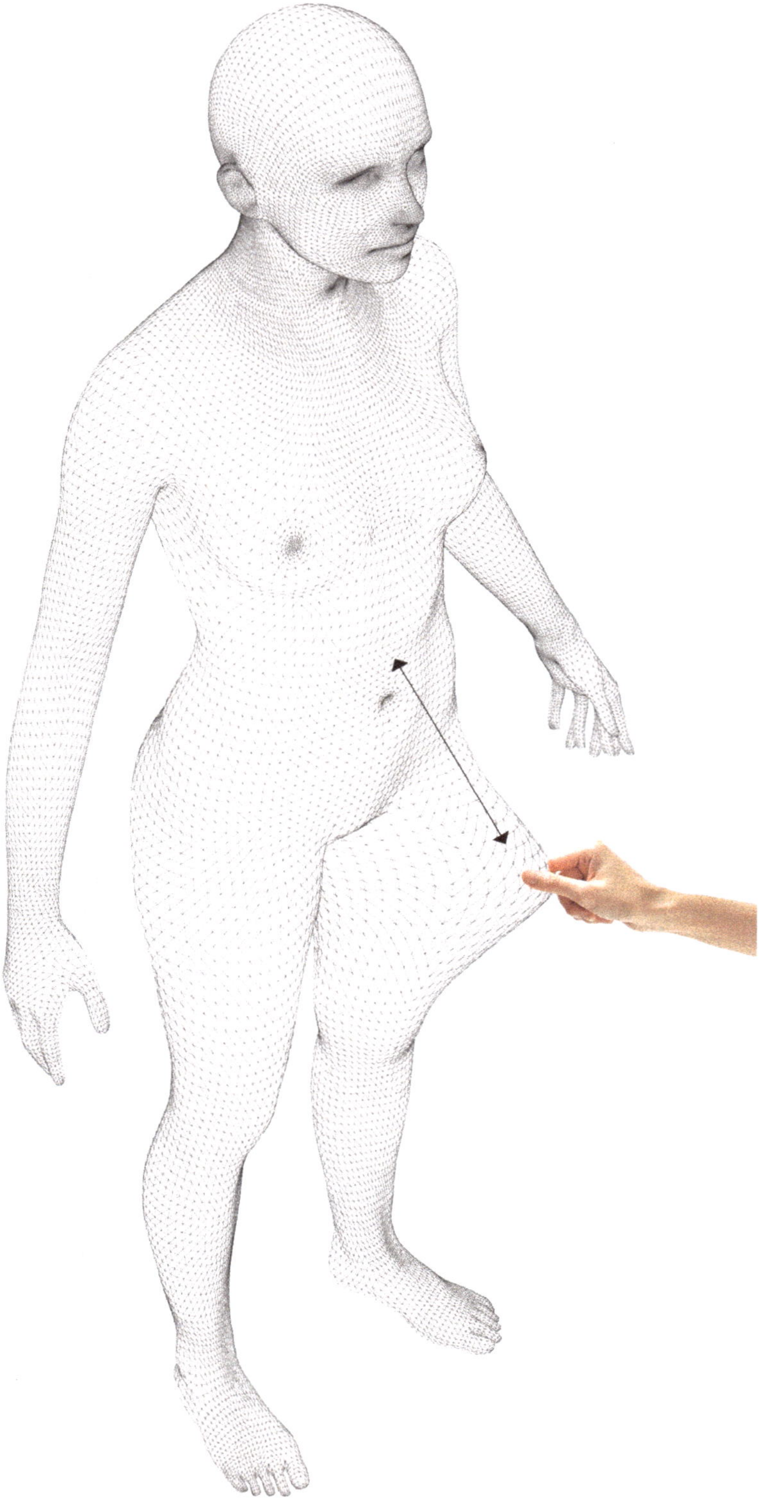

does. It puts its wearer at heightened risk of developing further injuries and health problems – as anyone who has ruptured their Achilles tendon, broken ribs, has a frozen shoulder, has recently had abdominal surgery, or plays professional sport well knows.

Tight spots and pull-strain lines can effectively shrink, tether or twist the LWS, changing the way this fleshy garment fits over the bones. This can, for instance, compress the joints between bones and may be a factor in their becoming worn and damaged. It may also pull the bones out of their normal position and the skeleton away from its normal alignment, and alter the ways they (and the rest of the body) move.

Painful, fewer, reduced, and less energy efficient body movements can further disturb the body's metabolic and physiological functioning, growth, healing, and recovery processes. Squished or stretched cells, tissues, organs, and organ systems work differently than they normally do, when they are not being strained in this way, and may not work so well and may eventually become damaged or unhealthy.

A poorly fitting LWS may also squash or abnormally stretch nerves, sensitive nerve endings, and even the brain and spinal cord. This can be painful. It can also affect the ways the nervous system senses, conducts, processes, and responds to sensory stimuli and information input.

Tight spots and pull-strain lines in certain parts of the LWS can also block or alter the normally free-flowing circulation of body fluids (e.g., blood, lymph, interstitial fluid, cerebrospinal fluid) – hence interfere with their nutritive, waste removal, immune defence, communicative, and healing roles. They can also be a factor in the LWS becoming abnormally congested and swollen with water, or oedematous. This type of swelling is most often seen in the feet, ankles, wrists and face, though it can occur almost anywhere – "No part is exempt; even the brain, heart, lungs, liver, stomach and bowels, bladder, kidneys, uterus, lymphatics, glands, nerves, veins, arteries, skin and all membranes are subject to swellings" (Still, 1899, p. 172). Oedema can be uncomfortable when it is accompanied by stiff and heavy limbs, cramping, headaches, or stomach bloating. It may also be life threatening – e.g., when it enters the lungs and makes it difficult to breathe, or fills up the head and squashes the brain.

If the tight spots and pull-strain lines are left alone and untreated, some will disappear by themselves – especially if the LWS's wearer is well-hydrated, healthy and gets plenty of non-injurious exercise. In many people, however, tight spots generally tend to hang around and accumulate, while the LWS slowly but surely becomes stiffer and less comfortable to wear. It gets injured, possibly again and again. It hurts. It doesn't move as well as it used to.

Before long, the body doesn't hum with its usual vitality, or work as effectively as it's meant to. It is less able to adapt to changes in its internal and outside conditions. It is less able to deal with and to recover from the wear and tear of everyday life. It hurts more and more often. It is less able to protect itself against illness. It doesn't heal as well as it used to. Yet it doesn't have to stay this way!

The LWS's wearer (and, unfortunately, also some of the health-care professionals they consult) may be completely unaware of their tight spots' existence and significance. They may not realise that these tight spots might be associated with the LWS wearer's other, more visible health problems – especially those that are complex, those that haven't been helped by conventional treatment (like Kahu's headache), and those that have lingered on way too long and become chronic (e.g., back and neck pain, swollen legs, breathing problems). They may instead think that they are just starting to 'feel their age,' and (sadly, quite wrongly) that there's nothing much that they or anyone else can do about this. Fortunately, as is explained in the next chapter, *there are many things that can be done by others*, and *that we can do ourselves* to help our LWSs stay well, eliminate their tight spots, ease their pain, and recover their functioning and health.

"Fascial strains can slowly tighten, causing the body to lose its physiologic adaptive capacity. Over time, the tightness spreads like a pull in a sweater or stocking. Flexibility and spontaneity of movement are lost, setting up the body for more trauma, pain, and limitation of movement. These powerful fascial restrictions begin to pull the body out of its three-dimensional alignment with the vertical gravitation axis, causing biomechanically inefficient, highly energy-consuming movement and posture." *(Barnes, 1990, p. 17)*

Healing the Living Wetsuit

Anna's elbow

Seven-year-old 'Anna' and her mother 'Jo'[24] were on the driveway talking to my next-door neighbor just as I arrived home. Jo, a former patient of mine, waved me over and introduced me to Anna, who was standing silently beside her. Jo explained that Anna had broken her arm bone (or humerus) just above the elbow a couple of months ago, when she fell from a tree she'd been climbing.

Fortunately, there'd been no complications, and no need for surgery. Her treatment had consisted of wearing a cast, which extended between her wrist and shoulder, for six weeks while the bone mended. The bone had healed well. So well, that Anna's hospital doctor, whom they'd last met ten days ago, had sent them away saying there was no need for any more follow-up visits. Her barely-any elbow movement, he said, would gradually return by itself during the next 12 months without any extra treatment. Jo told me she was concerned. She wasn't convinced by his reassurance that all was well when it clearly was not. The bone may have healed, but Anna and her elbow most definitely had not. Anna was unusually withdrawn and miserable, not at all like her normal high-spirited self. She could barely move her

24 Not their real names.

arm and elbow, and also wouldn't let anyone touch them. Could I suggest anything they could do to help Anna feel better, and to hopefully speed up her recovery?

The circumstances of our driveway meeting didn't allow me to perform a formal assessment, but I could see Anna was cradling her arm close to her chest, and protectively hunching her body over it. With Jo's help, she showed me how far she could, very cautiously, bend and straighten her firmly flexed elbow. Which was barely at all – at best, about 20 degrees, or 15% of its normal movement range. Anna said she couldn't move it any further because it hurt her to do so. When I asked her to show me where exactly it hurt, she pointed to several hard and sore lumps in the muscles above and below the front of her elbow.

My initial impression was that Anna had experienced a lot of pain since she'd injured her arm, and was now afraid of doing anything, or allowing anyone else to do anything, that might hurt her some more. This was a problem, as it was important to get her body moving normally as quickly as possible. A stiff elbow would make it difficult for her to do all of the things she ordinarily did – such as getting dried and dressed after a shower, eating with a knife and fork, getting in and out of the car with her schoolbag. Also, as a physio, I was quietly concerned about the safety of her running around and playing with other children while she had such a stiff arm. Another fall could have serious consequences.

I told Jo and Anna that it looked like her arm was healing really well, and that its normal movement would almost certainly return – just as the doctor had said it would. In response to Jo's question, I said I knew of something special that Anna could do that might help speed up her recovery. It was something she could do all by herself and didn't require anyone else's input. She would be in charge of this stage of her healing.

The something special was giving Anna a 'magic stone' and teaching her how to use it. I explained that our bodies are a lot like skeletons wearing wetsuits. She liked this idea, and 'got it' straightaway. It made sense to her and she could feel how the pain and stiffness in her arm were connected to some tight and sore spots in her wetsuit sleeve. Next, Anna chose a small river-smoothed stone from my garden (one that she liked the look of). Then I taught her how she could use it to gently press into and massage the pesky tight spots, so she could get rid of them without it hurting. Anna promptly tried this out on one of the tight spots and soon found that it was okay when she was the person doing the touching and pressing. She also noticed how her arm was now feeling more comfortable and was already a bit easier to move.

All of the above took less than ten minutes, yet the child I said good-bye to looked quite different to the child I'd met. Anna was now standing up straighter and was more cheerful. She now knew there was something she could do to help her arm feel better. I haven't seen her again, though Jo rang me several weeks later to say Anna and her elbow were both doing well. Anna appeared to have really enjoyed using her special stone right from the start. Jo had noticed her using it while quietly sitting watching television, and thought she'd also been using it while snuggled up safe and warm in her bed. Putting Anna in charge of treating her own arm, as and when it suited her, seemed to have been a happy success.

Bodywork

Every healthcare practitioner's understanding of human anatomy shapes their ideas about the ways bodies work, what happens when their patients' bodies are hurt or unwell, and what may be rationally done to protect and improve their patients' health. Thinking about the body as a skeleton wearing a fascia-pervaded LWS is obviously going to lead into the practitioner using some

LWS- and-fascia-relating treatment methods. Likewise, thinking about a body that is hypothetically lacking its fascial stroma will be associated with some quite different types of treatment. Both ways of conceptualising and caring for people's bodies are valuable and useful, even if we are only familiar with one of them. Neither, however, is, on its own, going to help everybody all of the time.

Fascia- and LWS-relating health care is explicitly concerned with the whole-body structure as well as the parts of it that are most obviously hurting, damaged, or diseased. As a result, this whole-body approach to treatment is generally known as bodywork. The overall goals of LWS-relating bodywork therapy basically are: (1) to find and help get rid of the tight spots that are presently upsetting a particular person's body's structural equilibrium, functioning and health; (2) to support that person's LWS's inherent ability to return to a more comfortable and healthy condition; and then (3) to teach that person about some of the things they themselves could easily do to care for and improve the health of their own LWS.

Bodywork practitioners (bodyworkers) are, on the whole, experts in tracking down and dealing with LWS tight spots. They collectively use a varying mix of reasonably natural and low-tech healing tools – including heating, cooling, mindful touch, massage, breathing techniques, stretching, compressing, rocking, vibrating, dry needling, energy techniques, myofascial cupping, mindful movement and exercise – to promote their clients' health and wellbeing (see Table 9.1). Much of what bodyworkers do can be used as a stand-alone form of professional treatment, though their work is more often than not used in conjunction with some other types of health care (e.g., nutritional advice, medical care, and or some other types of bodywork and movement therapy). Each course of treatment, and every treatment within that course, is tailored to meet both the immediate and long-term needs of a particular client (a LWS wearer). This is because a person's body is not a machine. It is not exactly the same as anyone else's body, and may not be the same as it was at the end of its last treatment session. While this individualised approach is usually pretty good for the person concerned, this lack of therapeutic standardisation has made it tricky to scientifically verify the results on a large scale.[25]

A simple way of understanding the bodywork way of doing things is to think of the LWS as the backdrop for a crime scene. The victim (e.g., the part of the body that is hurting) makes a lot of noise, loudly calling attention to its hurt and distress. Meanwhile, the gang of villains (felonious tight spots) lurk quietly hidden from view, unchecked and ready to cause more trouble in the future. In this way, a pain in the shoulder (victim) may have been triggered, for instance, by a scar in the arm, a tethered gall bladder, and or a troublesome tight spot deep in the leg.

The person with the sore shoulder might swallow some pain-killing tablets, rub some anti-inflammatory cream on their skin, and take things easy for a few days. Or, if the pain is really bad, their arm can't move properly, or they have reached the end of their tether with their body's continual series of injury complaints, they may decide to get some expert help.

There are many different types of professional helpers they might choose from – including acupuncturists, chiropractors, massage therapists, medical doctors, osteopaths, Pilates instructors, physiatrists, physiotherapists, surgeons, yoga therapists – all of whom have lots of experience with treating sore shoulders. Each helper's way of doing this is (as you now know) linked to their particular way of understanding of the body's, including its shoulder's, anatomical structure.

25 Randomised controlled trials are designed to test pharmaceutical medicines but are not suited to testing the efficacy of bodywork. The latter is generally better served by other types of research (e.g., mixed methods research studies).

In general, health practitioners who use the traditional, anatomised body model are likely to focus on identifying and fixing the loudly protesting 'victim' parts of the shoulder – such as the acromioclavicular joint, supraspinatus tendon, or subacromial bursa.

Many fascia- and LWS-relating practitioners will initially do this too, especially when the 'victim' body part is very sore, acutely inflamed, or physically damaged. Ensuring their patient's comfort and safety is usually their first and most pressing priority. Yet, once this has been done, they are unlikely to stop there. From their whole-body-encompassing viewpoint, they will almost certainly also want to consider whether their patient's symptoms might in some way be linked to the presence of a few cunningly concealed tight spots.

Tight spots seldom hang around at the crime scene waiting to be noticed. They, and the pull-strain lines that branch out from them, usually need to be deliberately sought out, found … and eliminated. This is important, as just treating the 'victim' on its own far too often fails to produce a good long-term result. It can be a bit like playing a game of medical whack-a-mole – i.e., separately fixing each symptom wherever it 'randomly' crops up. Sadly, this narrowly focused, problem-by-problem approach often only achieves a temporary improvement. This is illustrated, for example, in the elite athletes and sports people who sustain one injury after another, despite receiving an enormous amount of specialised professional help with separately fixing each of their injuries.

Table 9.1
Examples of bodywork treatment modalities

Some of the many presently available forms of practitioner-administered bodywork therapy that may be used (separately, or together) to help improve the health of the LWS, and its wearer. Information about them all is available on the Internet.

Acupuncture	Feldenkrais Method	Shiatsu
Craniosacral therapy	Myofascial Cupping	Structural Integration
Jing Method	Myofascial Release Therapy	Visceral Manipulation
Fascial Kinetics	ScarWork	Watsu Aquatic Therapy
Fascial Manipulation	Trager Approach	Yoga Therapy
Fascial Stretch Therapy	Trigger Point Therapy	Zero Balancing

A professional bodywork treatment typically involves most of the following series of happenings, some or all of which may be fitted in to one treatment session:

- Listening to the patient's story about what's bothering them, establishing their history and the series of events that have led them to ask for your help, medical test results and diagnoses, who they've already worked with, other treatments and outcomes.

- Looking at, for example, the way they hold and move their bodies as they enter and are in the room, their skin condition and colour, and their breathing rate.

- Manually palpating the LWS fabric to feel if it is denser, thicker, thinner, warmer, cooler, thicker, more swollen or tender than normal. Notice if it is puckered, twisted, stuck down, moving or not moving in certain directions.

- Identifying the LWS's problem areas, ascertaining their nature and severity, deciding on the local and global treatment that is required, and the order in which it ought to be done.

- Soothing the most distressing symptoms.

- Softening and eliminating troublesome tight spots.

- Stretching out and releasing the pull-strain lines that have radiated out from the troublesome tight spots.

- Helping to improve and readjust the way the LWS fits over the skeleton of bones that are embedded within so that the body as a whole may regain its normal, balanced state and be optimally aligned with Earth's gravity field.

- Helping improve the strength and condition of the LWS in order to assist the return of its (and the cells, tissues, organs and organ systems that are contained within its fleshy fabric) normal functioning and health.

- Educating the LWS's wearer about the LWS and bodywork, the assessment findings, the treatment, homework, self-care, health improvement, and future trouble prevention.

- Referring the LWS's wearer on to other types of health care provider if and when necessary.

- Monitoring and reassessing before, during, and after each treatment session.

"If fascia has tightened and is creating symptoms distant from the injury, all of the appropriate localized treatments will produce poor or temporary results because the imbalance and excess pressure from the myofascial tightness remain untreated." *(Barnes, 1990, p. 18)*

Self-care

As a fascia- and LWS-relating bodywork therapist, I consider my main role to be a *healing facilitator* rather than just a tight-spot problem fixer. Obviously, I and my many hundreds of thousands, if not millions, of international bodywork colleagues do what we do to directly help ease our patient's difficulties. Despite this, a large and perhaps equally important part of our work is educative – i.e., teaching people about what they may do to help themselves, and, when applicable, what they might do to help each other (e.g., their child or spouse).

All of my patients get given some LWS-benefitting home-work – i.e., at least one thing they could do at home to boost the benefit of their professional treatment session(s) and to help themselves heal. None of them are compelled to do this, yet most of them do it because they want to feel better as soon as they possibly can. Over the years, their comments have made it clear that they appreciate being shown some simple, down-to-earth things they can do to help themselves, without spending much, if any, money.

Each person's homework is tailored to fit their health needs, their self-care treatment preferences, and the resources they have at hand. The same one homeworky task is unlikely to be suitable for everybody and may not be right for a person at different stages of their recovery. We discuss and design their homework together, as it is important to ensure it is something that they are comfortable with and can see themselves doing. The homework-doer must also clearly understand the linkage between their LWS problem and their given task. They are going to be doing the work, so they need to know the whys and wherefores, and how to do whatever it is properly and safely.

My instructions focus on equipping that person to help themselves this way, and seldom contain any hard and fast rules about 'how much', and 'how often' as I want to encourage that person to find out what works best for them. Whatever they do, however, must definitely not involve them inflicting any strain or pain on their body. The old 'no pain, no gain' saying has absolutely no place in this type of treatment approach due to the very real risk that it can cause harm to the LWS and its human wearer.

Some of the many homeworky things I might suggest to my patients include, for example:

- Going for a walk most days
- Monitoring and improving their posture
- Monitoring and improving their breathing
- Applying a hot pack
- Self-massage

- Mindful stretching
- Dry skin brushing
- Making sure they drink enough water
- Getting enough sleep, and
- Maybe using a stone to smooth away some of their own tight spots … just like Anna.

There are many excellent reasons for doing LWS-homework that, depending on the person concerned, might help them to help themselves:

- Get rid of their tight spots, and pull-strain lines
- Lessen pain and inflammation
- Reduce fluid congestion and swelling
- Speed up and progress their recovery from their current health problem
- Make it easier for them to move and do the things they want to do
- Make it easier for them to breathe
- Lessen their anxiety and stress
- Improve their sleep
- Improve their general health and wellbeing
- Enhance their creativity and productivity at work
- Physically strengthen their body
- Boost their athletic performance and competitiveness
- Lessen their need to seek other forms of expensive and time-consuming professional treatment
- Help themselves manage their body's pain and discomfort while waiting for a medical diagnosis or specialised medical or surgical treatment
- Help themselves manage their body's pain and discomfort while confined at home during a global disease pandemic.

The Living Wetsuit in the 21st Century

An unexpected wake-up call

I've often felt like I am being guided through my life by something bigger than me. I know this is not particularly unusual, as many other people feel like this too. Sometimes it feels like I've been lifted by the scruff of the neck and am being quietly encouraged to move in a new direction – in much the same way a mother cat lifts and shifts one of her kittens. Just when I'm comfortably puttering along with life, I seem to get dealt a new hand to play with. One of these times was when my twin sons were 12 years old. I felt this strong urge to take them out of school for a few months and travel around the world. It was crazy but it somehow happened. It changed their lives, and it changed mine too.

During our round-the-world adventure, we spent a few delightful days with some American friends who lived in Boston. One of them, Laura, had suffered a serious whiplash injury after a car crash. Despite having been seen by several highly respected medical doctors, and done everything they said she ought to do, Laura was still unwell and in pain nearly a year later. By then she was feeling pretty desperate about her lack of recovery, so when a friend suggested she go and see a physical therapist who specialised in a new form of treatment called craniosacral therapy

(CST),[26] she decided to give it a go. To her surprise, CST helped her straight away. She couldn't say what happened, or why it had worked. The main thing, as far as she was concerned, was that it had soon fixed all of her car crash-related health problems.

When Laura told me this story I felt an unaccountably urgent need to meet her seemingly miracle-working physical therapist. Thankfully, the therapist ignored her several-months-long waiting list and agreed to see me for an hour the following day. We sat down and talked for most of this time, and I then lay down on her treatment table for ten minutes so she could show me what CST felt like. I didn't feel anything special happen, which I later learned is pretty normal with this type of treatment, but I knew straightway that something inside me had changed. I couldn't put my finger on what it was. I somehow just knew that I needed to learn a lot more about CST, even though it wasn't then being taught in my home country. Life was grabbing me by the scruff of the neck again. "What on the earth's going on here?" I thought to myself. I'd had no idea CST even existed before we'd visited our friends. And, for goodness sake, people don't just pack up their bags and flit off overseas to study this sort of stuff – well, not the sorts of people I knew. Yet I knew with every fibre of my being that it was something I needed to do, even though it made absolutely no sense to me then.

A few short months later I returned to America. My first four-day Upledger Institute CST course was in San Francisco. I remember I had a headache most of the time because I was trying so hard to understand everything my classmates and I were being taught. The CST teaching was based on a new way of thinking about the body's structure. I'd previously been taught about a body that was mostly made of muscles and bones. My CST teachers spoke about these, but they also spoke about something called fascia. Fascia is important, so they said, because it is spread all through the body and connects everything in it

26 Craniosacral therapy (CST) is a gentle, hands-on approach to evaluating and improving many health conditions that grew out of American osteopathic physician John E. Upledger's observation of a rhythmic pulsation of the membranous covering of the spinal cord (between six and twelve cycles per minute) when assisting with a spinal surgical operation during the early 1970s. His 1975–1983 employment as a professor of biomechanics, at Michigan State University's College of Osteopathic Medicine, enabled him and a team of anatomists, physiologists, biophysicists, and bioengineers to investigate this pulse, and to consider its clinical significance.

together. *Fascial restrictions*[27] – places where the fascia has tightened and lost its normal ability to move – inhibit fascia's normal extensibility and ability to move freely. The tension emanating from these tight spots could be transmitted elsewhere in the body via its three-dimensional web of fascial tissue, and then give rise to some other new sets of problems and symptoms. CST works, they explained, by very gently releasing tight spots in the fascia and stopping other things in the body (including the brain, spinal cord, and nerves) from being squashed and injured. All of this was quite foreign to me, yet I was determined to wrap my mind around it. I already knew that this new way of thinking about treating people's bodies was really important.

On the third day of the course we were shown a video that showcased the work of the Upledger Clinic in Florida. This is a place where people travel to from all over the world to be treated by a team of highly trained health professionals who use CST in their work. This video showed how CST was providing relief and hope for people with conditions that hadn't been helped by other more conventional forms of treatment (some of whom had been medically dismissed as lost causes). It also showed people with ordinary conditions who were recovering faster and better than anything I was used to seeing, and some who were choosing to use it as a means of improving their health and sense of wellbeing. Much to my embarrassment, tears streamed down my face. Tears of wonder. Tears of relief that such a place existed. Tears of joy to have discovered another way of being able to help people improve and recover their health. This new and different style of treatment felt so right and important that I knew I was going to have to do something about raising people's awareness of it in my own country.

When I came back to New Zealand, I started incorporating CST in my physiotherapy practice. My patients now got better faster than they generally used to, and often improved in ways I hadn't expected. Long standing pain frequently disappeared

27   Another name for LWS tight spots.

after one treatment. Bodies and the joints between their bones straightened out and moved better. Teeth knocked loose and blackened by injury became stable again and recovered their normal vitality and colour. Distressed and colicky babies settled and slept peacefully. Irritable infants, and their frazzled parents, recovered their equanimity and good humour. Squashed nerves were freed from whatever was squashing them without surgical intervention. People with whiplash and head injuries made astonishing recoveries. The people I worked with, their families, the growing number of doctors who referred them, and myself were amazed and delighted by the results of this new fascia-relating way of working. Something really good and worthwhile was clearly happening, even if none of us fully understood the reasons for it.

It didn't take long before I realised that I needed to spread the good news and the idea of deliberately working with fascia with my colleagues, so that they too (and hopefully their patients) might experience its benefits. The question was how best to do this?

Like John Upledger before me, I soon found I could personally only treat a certain number of people, so could only influence a relatively small number of people this way. I needed to find some other ways of doing this. Ways that would spread these new ideas further, like the ripples spreading out from a stone dropped into a pond of still water. The first thing I could do was to further my education and learn as much as I could about CST and possibly some other types of fascia-relating bodywork treatment. I also needed to find out what different groups of student healthcare professionals were being taught about anatomy and fascia.[28] If my experience to date was anything to go by, it was possible that some of them were learning diddly squat about fascia and its centrality in health care. I went deep with my studies. I travelled overseas to attend courses. I sponsored teachers to come to New Zealand. I taught courses myself. Much to my surprise, I even earned some university qualifications. Some of my colleagues and family members were initially sceptical, and at times dismissive, of what I was doing. Some of them still are. In the long run their negative responses made me more determined than ever to continue doing what I was doing, and see if I could help spread some of the things I'd been learning about fascia and fascia-relating health care further out into the world. Both are simply too important to ignore!

Knowledge is powerful

So why does our knowledge of fascia actually matter? Especially as lots of people, including many health professionals, have so far lived most of their lives knowing very little, if anything, about it.

It matters because knowledge is powerful. Knowledge helps us understand and explain things. It is used to justify certain courses of action. It gives us authority, the power to choose and make decisions. Knowledge, whatever it is about, is multifaceted, and it is continuously evolving. New knowledge is a tool that makes it possible for us to understand and do things we could not have previously considered thinking and doing.

Anatomy is a type of knowledge that helps us understand the body's structural makeup. Anatomical knowledge is a powerful tool because it helps people understand their bodies' structure. This in turn makes it possible for them to also understand:

- How their bodies normally develop, grow, and perform their work,
- How and why these things change when their bodies are affected by injury and disease, and
- What can best be done to protect, maintain, and improve their health.

In other words, our knowledge of anatomy powerfully influences the choices we can make about our bodies' health care. None of us can afford, as Melanchthon once stated (see p. 40), "to rest in ignorance of the structure of [our] own body", especially when our knowledge of it shapes the ways we are able to think about looking after it and helping it heal.

Having a simple, yet up-to-date and well-grounded knowledge of our body's living form can help us become more self-reliant in matters concerning our own health. It boosts our authority and enables us to have more say-so (and, if we want it, more control) over our own health and health care decisions, than if we chose to remain ignorant on this subject.

If it is taught well, lay people can easily learn some anatomy. It does not have to be complicated and difficult. Unless we are planning on becoming health professionals, most of us can manage pretty well without mastering all of anatomy's scientific language and details. We can, when needs be, check out some of the finer details on Google. We can also call in some extra help from our professional health helpers – keeping in mind that some of them may well have some gaps in their anatomical knowledge of the living and whole human body, its fascia, and fascia-relating health care!

Upgrading our knowledge of anatomy and fascia is worthwhile. It helps us make some better-informed choices about the ways we look after and remedially treat our own bodies, and hopefully improve their health and wellness. It may also help us become more effective in helping the people we are responsible for caring for – such as our family members, employees, or patients. Doing this may or may not increase our/their use of fascia-relating bodywork and movement therapies. It may or may not help lessen our society's extensive use of high-tech medicines and surgery. The latter are unquestionably of great value, especially when dealing with acute and infectious medical conditions. Yet they also have some important shortcomings:

- They can cost a lot of money
- They aren't available to everyone, everywhere, and all of the time
- They have limited success with many long-term health problems
- They may not be compatible with some people's belief systems (e.g., vaccination, blood transfusions, gene therapy)
- And they can sometimes cause harm – to people, to animals, and to the environments we cohabit.

As with any other form of knowledge, the world's knowledge of anatomy and fascia is continually developing and evolving. During the past few decades there has been a large and well-documented resurgence of interest in fascia. It seems like fascia has suddenly stepped out into the limelight after an extended period of "a Cinderella-like neglect" (Klinger & Schleip, 2015, p. 3). The ways fascia is now being seen and understood in the world have moved on from the ways it was known in the past.

It is possible that our world has reached yet another tipping point in all sorts of ways we understand and do things (perhaps even on par with the scale of change expressed during the European Renaissance). It is possible that humanity is once again being pressed to make a profound and momentous shift forwards in its thinking. It could be that the time has come for us to collectively evolve and become better, and better-informed, humans. For this to happen, we must make some fundamental changes – like taking better care of the bodies and the environments we live in, to work more collaboratively and fairly, to live more peaceably together. Tipping points and paradigm shifts such as these don't happen overnight. They are associated with an enormous cascade of smaller (though not small) related happenings in our everyday worlds. One of these could well be something as simple as learning about our bodies' whole and alive structure – not just its dead and dissected one. One that recognises the importance of fascia and the energies that enliven it. Doing this could help us broaden our knowledge of our bodies and their anatomy, and in turn increase the number of ways we might commonsensically improve our health and wellbeing. History shows that this type of change is likely to be far reaching and long-lasting in effect.[29]

The LWS and the world

The idea of a skeleton wearing a LWS is a simple and fun way of explaining the body's structure that, my experience has shown me, instantly makes sense to most people. More than that, it provides them with a short and sweet set of well-grounded and up-to-date anatomical knowledge that they can use to help them make and act on their own healthcare decisions.

Behind the scenes, the LWS body model incorporates everything that anatomists have learned to date about our body's anatomised structural form … then adds some more to it. The LWS is a highly practical and up-to-date way of conceptualising the natural structure of people's bodies, our bodies – i.e., bodies that are whole and alive rather than dead and dissected. Bodies that naturally contain lots of fascia and are infused with life-endowing energy. The LWS model is academically robust,[30] yet people don't need to have a fancy education to understand it. This all sounds pretty good, but it seriously needs to be like this so that everybody – not just those with specialised university degrees and professional health care jobs – can take better care of their own and each other's bodies.

Adding fascia back into our knowledge of anatomy effectively increases the number of ways we may be able to do this, some of which may well be:

29 This conclusion is based on the concept of a discontinuous progression in the development of knowledge explicated by Michel Foucault (1926–1984), a French philosopher and historian of ideas (summarised in Gutting, 2005).

30 At least as solid as its widely used dead and fascia-less counterparts.

- Safer for people and animals, and the environments we all live in
- Less expensive in terms of our time and money
- More closely aligned to our personal, cultural, and ethical beliefs and values
- More accessible and sustainable to us than what is currently on offer
- Complements and perhaps boosts the effectiveness of the other forms of treatment we may already be using.

Poor health does not necessarily have to be a life sentence. Some health problems – especially the complex, painful and chronic ones – may seem like they are impossible to solve. In many instances, it can be helpful to look at them from a different anatomical perspective. It's never too late to turn many of them around or just make them more tolerable to live with.

It is highly likely that there are several things you may not have already thought of that *you* could safely and easily do to help you improve your health … all of which basically relate to your understanding of your body's anatomical structure. Self-care (in conjunction with conventional medical advice) is a useful form of treatment – especially when it allows you to care for your body in ways that you can financially afford, are congruent with your beliefs and values, are accessible (even when you're stuck at home during a pandemic), and can be fitted in to the way you live your life. Self-care is something you can nearly always turn and go to.

Our world is undergoing great change. For a variety of reasons, not everyone can rely on receiving as much high-tech professional health care as they would like. It may therefore be useful for all of us to learn some more ways we might use to help us care for our own and each other's health.

Attending to the comfort and health of your LWS is possibly far more important than you may have realised before reading this book, and may very well help make your body a healthier and much happier place to live in. Also, it could conceivably (and hopefully) delay or prevent your requiring some more drastic forms of medical and surgical treatment in times to come, and, should you go down that track, help speed up your recovery.

The Living Wetsuit is a person's whole, fascia-containing and life-energy-infused fleshy body garment. This modern anatomical analogy works because it is:

- Simple and full of common sense
- Easily understood by children and adults
- Stacks up academically
- Practical and useful
- Used by health professionals and health educators
- Used by health researchers and scientists
- Used by lay people as a tool that helps them have more control over managing their own health and health care
- Has genuine potential to help solve some of human society's most pressing and difficult-to-solve population health problems.

Further Information

Discover some simple, everyday things that you can do to take care of, and hopefully help improve the comfort and health of your Living Wetsuit by downloading your free copy of the ebook, *A Basic 6-Point Maintenance Guide for Living Wetsuit Owners*, from:

www.sueadstrum.com/LWS-resources

 If you would like to learn more about anatomy, fascia, and the Living Wetsuit, please visit:

www.sueadstrum.com

Glossary

Anatomical adaptation	Change in structure of a body part that helps it adjust to changes in its current environment or workload
Adhesions	Bands of scar-like tissue that form between two internal body surfaces
Adipocyte	An adipose, or fat, cell
Adipose tissue	Tissue mainly composed of adipocyte cells
Anatomy	The scientific art of describing the body's structure A bioscientific occupational profession that describes the body's structure An internationally agreed-upon set of concepts and representations that bioscientifically describes the body's physical structure A formally taught curriculum subject that teaches students about the body's anatomical structure
Anatomies	Socio-culturally agreed-upon sets of concepts and representations that systematically describe the body's structure
Aponeurosis	A flat sheet of fibrous tissue connecting a muscle and the part it moves
Arteries	Blood vessels that conduct blood away from the heart
Arteriole	A small-diameter branch of an artery
Axon	The long, electrical impulse conducting part of a nerve cell (neuron)
Biotensegrity	Biological tensegrity. Application of tensegrity principles to biological structures, including human bodies

Bodywork	A general term for a raft of whole-body centred treatment methods and techniques that varyingly use a mix of heating, cooling, mindful touch, massage, breath, stretching, compressing, rocking, vibrating, dry needling, energy, movement and exercise to promote a person's health and wellbeing. May be used as an adjunctive or stand-alone form of treatment
Bodyworker	A bodywork therapy practitioner
Bursa (plural, bursae)	A small, fluid-filled sac that helps reduce friction between some moving body parts
Cadaver	A dead body, or corpse
Capillaries	The smallest blood vessels that form a network between the arterioles and venules
Cell	The smallest biological structural unit
Collagen	A strong fibrous protein that is abundantly found in fascia. Most abundant protein in human body
Congenital	In existence at birth
Contractile	Capable of contraction
Craniosacral therapy	A fascia-relating system of bodywork therapy that uses light touch to help release deep tensions in the body, eliminate pain, restore movement, and improve health and wellbeing
Culture	An integrated and integrating social environment characterised by shared philosophies, practices, and attitudes
Dehydration	Loss or removal of water
Deep fascia	Dense fibrous fascia that surrounds and interpenetrates muscles and groups of muscles
Elastin	An elastic protein
Embalming	Preserving a dead body with chemicals to protect it from decay
Endomysium	Fascial substance ensheathing each and every muscle fibre
Epimysium	The dense fascial sheath of a muscle

Extracellular	Outside the cell
Extracellular matrix	Material produced by cells and excreted to extracellular space in tissue. Contains a mix of extracellular structural protein fibres and ground substance
Fascia	The body's soft connective tissue parts
A fascia (plural, fasciae)	A macroscopic piece of fascial tissue
Fascial entrapment neuropathy	A group of nerve disorders (including carpal tunnel syndrome) caused by chronic compression or stretching of nerves by the fascia that adjoins them
Fascia-relating bodywork modality	A system of bodywork treatment that overtly relates to the treatment of fascia
Fascial substance	Fascial ground substance
Fascial system	A body-pervading web of fascial tissue that takes shape in a variety of functional formats
Fascial tissue	Soft, collagen-containing, connective tissue
Fasciatome	A section of deep fascia supplied by the same nerve root
Fibroblasts	Cells that make and maintain fascial extracellular matrix
Fulcrum	A fixed point around which two arms of a lever rotate
Granulation tissue	New fascial (connective) tissue with many capillaries in it. Found at edges of healing wounds
Ground substance	The amorphous gel-like substance that connective tissue cells and fibres are set in
Health profession	A paid occupational vocation that requires prolonged training and a formal qualification
Health practitioner	A person practicing a particular healing discipline (e.g., massage, medicine)

| **Histology** | A branch of anatomy that studies the microscopic structure of tissues and organs |

Histology — A branch of anatomy that studies the microscopic structure of tissues and organs

Holistic — Perceiving something as a whole unit

Inflammation — A body's defensive response to tissue injury

Inflammatory exudate — Fluid that leaks out of blood vessels into areas of inflamed tissue

Interstitial fluid — Fluid around cells

Ion — An atom or molecule with a positive or negative charge

Joint — An articular junction between two bones

Lever system — A machine in which the application of mechanical force (*effort*) causes two rigid bars (*levers*) to move in relation to each other around a fixed point, or *fulcrum*

Ligaments — Bands of dense, Type 1 collagen-reinforced fascia that connect bones, or support visceral organs

Lymph — Protein-rich fluid that flows through the lymphatic vessels

Lymphatic vessels — Tubes that collect lymph from tissues and return it to the blood circulatory system

Lymphocyte — A type of small immune cell found in lymphatic fluid, spleen and lymph nodes

Macrophage — A type of large immune cell that engulfs and digests harmful bacteria and microbes, cancer cells, cellular debris, and other foreign substances

Macroscopic — Visible to the naked eye

Manual therapy — Body treatment physically administered with a therapist's hands. Also known as 'hands-on treatment'

Mast cell — A type of immune cell in connective tissue

Microscopic — So small that can only be seen with the aid of a microscope

Mind-body therapy — Treatment techniques that positively affect the physical and mental aspects of a person's body

Model — A way of thinking about something (such as the body)

Molecule	A chemical particle consisting of two or more chemically-joined atoms
Movement therapy	Therapeutic use of body movement to positively affect a person's (physical and or mental) health
Muscle fibre	A muscle cell
Muscle spindle	A stretch sensitive receptor in skeletal muscle
Myofascia	Combination of muscle (*myo-*) and fascia (*fascia*)
Myofascial chain (myofascial meridian)	A longitudinally connected string of myofascial and fascial structures
Myofascial Release Therapy	A myofascia-relating system of bodywork therapy that uses gentle sustained pressure to help release deep tensions in the body. eliminate pain, restore movement, and improve health and wellbeing
Nerve	A cable-like bundle of fascia-wrapped nerve fibres (axons)
Neuron	Nerve cell
Nutrients	Chemical substances absorbed from food that body uses for energy and cell building
Organ	A body part formed from two or more types of tissue and adapted to perform a certain function (e.g., the liver)
Organ system	A group of organs that work together to perform a particular set of body functions (e.g., the nervous system, the fascial system)
Organism	A living whole animal (e.g., a person)
Ossuary	A building where human bones are stored; charnel house
Osteoblasts	Bone forming cells
Osteoclasts	Cells that resorb and break down bone
Osteocytes	Mature bone cells
Parenchyma	Functionally specialised cells in an organ or tissue
Pathology	The scientific study of how the body and its parts are affected by injury and disease

Pericardium (pericardial sac)	Double-walled fascial sac surrounding the heart and the large blood vessels that enter and leave the heart
Perimysium	Fascia that encloses bundles (fasciculi) of muscle fibres
Physiology	The scientific study of how the body and its parts normally work
Plasma cell	A type of immune cell that makes antibodies
Pleura (plural, pleurae)	The double-walled fascial sac surrounding a lung
Professional health care	Ways people are paid to do to help look after and improve somebody else's health
Public health care	Ways people protect and promote community health
Rolfing® (or Structural Integration®)	A myofascia-relating system of bodywork therapy and movement education that helps release deep tensions in the body, eliminate pain, restore movement, and improve health and wellbeing. This bodywork treatment modality was initially developed by Ida Rolf, PhD
Sarcolemma	A membrane enveloping a muscle fibre (muscle cell)
Scar	An area of fibrous tissue that replaces normal skin or other tissue during the wound repair process
Sensory receptors	Information receptive endings of sensory nerve cells
Septum (pl. septa)	A dividing wall or partition
Skeletal muscle	A muscle that is connected to the skeleton. Composed of striped, multinucleated, cylindrical skeletal muscle cells
Social	Of or relating to human society
Stroma	The connective and supporting fascial tissue framework within an organ
Synovial joint	A synovial fluid-filled junction between two cartilage-tipped bones
Temporal	Of or pertaining to time
Tendons	Cords of dense Type 1 collagen-reinforced fascia that connect muscles to other body parts, especially bones

Tensegrity	Property of a mechanically stable three-dimensional structure built from isolated (non-contiguous bars or struts) components that are compressed within a continuous net of constantly tensioned cables
Tight spot	A place where the LWS fabric has become thicker, less pliable, and more tender than usual
Tipping point	The moment at which a series of small happenings set off a large and important change in the world
Tissue	A group of cells that have a similar structure and function together as a unit
Transdisciplinary research	An integrative research strategy that amalgamates science and humanities concepts and methods to holistically explore an issue that crosses several disciplinary boundaries
Veins	Blood vessels that transport blood towards the heart
Venule	A small vein
Visceral organs	Organs housed in the chest, abdomen and pelvis
White blood cell	A member of a family of immune cells that help body fight off infections

References

A

Adstrum, S. (2015). Fascial eponyms may help elucidate terminological and nomenclatural development. *Journal of Bodywork and Movement Therapies 19*(3): 516–525.

Adstrum, S., Hedley, G., Schleip, R., Stecco, C., & Yucesoy, C. A. (2017). Defining the fascial system. *Journal of Bodywork and Movement Therapies 21*(1): 173–177.

Adstrum, S., & Nicholson, H. (2019). A history of fascia. *Clinical Anatomy 23*(7): 862–870.

Agneessens, C. (2001). *The fabric of wholeness: Biological intelligence and relational gravity.* Aptos, CA: Quantum Institute, Inc.

B

Barnes, J. F. (1990). *Myofascial release: The search for excellence.* Paoli, PA: Myofascial Release Seminars.

Benias, P. C., Wells, R. G., Sackey-Abagye, B., Klaven, H., Reidy, J., Buonocore, D., Miranda, M., Kornacki S., Wayne M., Carr-Locke D. L., & Theise N. D. (2018). Structure and distribution of an unrecognized interstitium in human tissues. *Scientific Reports 8*: 4947.

Benor, D. J. (2004). *Consciousness, bioenergy and healing: Self-healing and energy medicine for the 21st century.* Medford, NJ: Wholistic Healing Publications.

Bichat, X. (1813). *A treatise on the membranes in general and on different membranes in particular* (J. G. Coffin, Trans.). Boston, MA: Cummings and Hilliard. [Original work published 1800]

Birke, L. (1999). *Feminism and the biological body.* Brunswick, NJ: Rutgers University Press.

Bordoni, B., & Simonelli, M. (2018). The awareness of the fascial system. *Cureus 10*(10): e3397. doi: 10.7759/cureus.3397

C

Crooke, H. (1615). *Mikrokosmographia: A description of the body of man together with the controversies and figures thereto belonging*. London, UK: William Iaggard.

Crooke, H. (1651). *Mikrokosmographia: A description of the body of man together with the controversies and figures thereto belonging* (2nd ed.). London, UK: John Clarke.

Crystal, D. (2011). *The story of English in 100 words*. London, UK: Profile Books.

G

Galeano, E. (1997). *Walking words* (M. Fried, Trans.). New York, NY: Norton. [Original work published 1993]

Gallaudet, B. B. (1931). *A description of the planes of fascia of the human body: With special reference to the fascia of the abdomen, pelvis and perineum*. New York, NY: Columbia University Press.

Gutting, G. (2005). *Foucault: A very short introduction*. Oxford, UK: Oxford University Press.

H

Heidegger, M. (1977). *The question concerning technology and other essays*. New York, NY: Harper & Row.

Huijing, P. A. (2009). Epimuscular myofascial force transmission: A historical review and implications for new research. International Society of Biomechanics Muybridge Award Lecture, Taipei, 2007. *Journal of Biomechanics 42*(1): 9–21.

J

Janssen, I., Heymsfield, S. B., Wang, Z., & Ross, R. (2000). Skeletal muscle mass and distribution in 468 men and women aged 18–88 yr. *Journal of Applied Physiology 89*(1): 81–88.

Jones, F. W. (1943). *Structure and function as seen in the foot*. London, UK: Ballière, Tindall and Cox.

K

Kaptchuk, T. J. (2000). *The web that has no weaver: Understanding Chinese medicine*. Chicago, IL: Contemporary Books.

Kern, M. (2001). *Wisdom in the body: The craniosacral approach to essential health*. Berkeley, CA: North Atlantic Books.

Klinger, W., & Schleip, R. (2015). Fascia as a body-wide tensional network: Anatomy, biomechanics and physiology. In Schleip, R., & Baker, A. (Eds.), *Fascia in sport and movement*. Pencaitland, UK: Handspring Publishers (pp. 3–11).

Koffka, K. (1935). *Principles of Gestalt psychology*. New York, NY: Harcourt, Brace & Co. https://archive.org/details/in.ernet.dli.2015.7888/page/n191/mode/2up?q=sum [accessed September 2020]

L

Lewis, J. (2012). *A. T. Still: From the dry bone to the living man*. Blaenau Ffestiniog, UK: Dry Bone Press.

Levin, S. M. (2006). Tensegrity: The new biomechanics. In Hudson, M., & Ellis, R. (Eds.), *Textbook of musculoskeletal medicine*. Oxford, UK: Oxford University Press (pp. 69–80).

M

Maitland, J. (1995). *Spacious body: Explorations in somatic ontology*. Berkeley, CA: North Atlantic Books.

Marieb, E. N., & Hoehn, K. (2019). *Human anatomy & physiology* (11th, global ed.). Harlow, UK: Pearson.

Montross, C. (2007). *Body of work*. New York, NY: Penguin Press.

Morens, D. M., & Taubenberger, J. K. (2011). Pandemic influenza: Certain uncertainties. *Reviews in Medical Virology 21*(5): 262–284.

Morens, D. M., North, J., & Taubenberger, J. K. (2010). Eyewitness accounts of the 1510 influenza pandemic in Europe. *Lancet 376*(9756): 1894–1895.

Murray, A. D. (2009). *Fascia*. Chicago, IL: The Green Lantern Press.

Myers, T. W. (2014). *Anatomy trains: Myofascial meridians for manual and movement therapists* (3rd ed.). Edinburgh, UK: Churchill Livingstone Elsevier.

N

Netter, F. H. (1997). *Atlas of human anatomy* (2nd ed.). East Hanover, NJ: Novartis.

Nicholls, D. A. (2018). *The end of physiotherapy*. London, UK: Routledge.

O

Oschman, J. L. (2012). Fascia as a body-wide communication system. In Schleip, R., Findley, T. W., Chaitow, L., & Huijing, P. A. (Eds.), *Fascia: The tensional network of the human body*. Edinburgh, UK: Churchill Livingstone Elsevier (pp. 103–110).

P

Paulus, S. (2013). The core principles of osteopathic philosophy. *International Journal of Osteopathic Medicine 16*(1): 11–16.

Paulus, S. (2009). *Life chronology of A. T. Still.* http://osteopathichistory.com/pagesside2/LifeChronology. html [accessed September 2020]

Pollack, G. H. (2001). *Cells, gels, and the engines of life: A new, unifying approach to cell function.* Seattle, WA: Ebner & Sons.

R

Roberts, A. (2021). *Cutting and Crisis – Rediscovering the human body* [Audio recording]. BBC Sounds. https:// www.bbc.co.uk/sounds/play/m000rd12 [accessed February 2021]

Rolf, I. P. (1977). *Rolfing: The integration of human structures.* Santa Monica, CA: Dennis-Landman.

S

Sawday, J. (1995). *The body emblazoned.* London, UK: Routledge.

Saxe, J. G. (1949). The blindmen and the elephant. From *Childcraft* (Vol. 2 of 14), *Storytelling and other poems* (pp. 122–123). Chicago, IL: Field Enterprises, Inc. [Original work published 1872]

Selzer, R. (1976). *Mortal lessons: Notes on the art of surgery.* New York, NY: Simon and Schuster.

Scarr, G. (2014). *Biotensegrity: The structural basis of life.* Pencaitland, UK: Handspring Publishing.

Schleip, R., Gabbiani, G., Wilke, J., Naylor, I., Hinz, B., Zorn, A., Jäger, H., Breul, R., Schreiner, S., & Klinger, W. (2019). Fascia is able to actively contract and may thereby influence musculoskeletal dynamics: A histo-chemical and mechanographic investigation. *Frontiers in Physiology 10*: 336.

Schleip, R., & Stecco, C. (2021). Fascia as sensory organ. In Schleip, R. (Ed.), *Fascia in sport and movement* (2nd ed.). Pencaitland, UK: Handspring Publishers.

Siraisi, N. G. (1995). Early anatomy in comparative perspective: Introduction. *Journal of the History of Medicine and Allied Sciences 50*(1): 3–10.

Standring, S. (2016a). A brief history of topographical anatomy. *Journal of Anatomy 229*(1): 32–62.

Standring, S. (Ed.). (2016b). *Gray's anatomy: The anatomical basis of clinical practice* (41st ed.). Edinburgh, UK: Churchill Livingstone.

Stecco, C., Adstrum, S., Hedley, G., Schleip, R., & Yucesoy, C. A. (2018). Update on fascial nomenclature. *Journal of Bodywork and Movement Therapies 22*(2): 354.

Stecco, C., Pavan, P. G., Porzionato, A., Macchi, V., Lancerotto, L., Carniel, E. L., & De Caro, R. (2009). Mechanics of crural fascia: From anatomy to constitutive modeling. *Surgical and Radiologic Anatomy 31*(7): 523–529.

Stecco, C., & Schleip, R. (2016). A fascia and the fascial system. *Journal of Bodywork and Movement Therapies 20*(1): 139–140.

Still, A. T. (1899). *Philosophy of osteopathy.* https://archive.org/stream/philosophyosteo00stilgoog#page/n10/mode/2up [accessed September 2020]

Stilwell, D. L. (1957). Regional variations in the innervation of deep fasciae and aponeuroses. *Anatomical Record 127*(4): 635–653.

T

Tanaka, G., & Kawamura, H. (1992). *Reference man models based on normal data from human populations* (Report No. 23). Report of the Task Group on Reference Man, The International Commission on Radiological Protection. https://www.irpa.net/irpa10/cdrom/00602.pdf [accessed November 2020]

Thompson, T. (1852). *Annals of influenza, or epidemic catarrhal fever in Great Britain. From 1510–1837.* London, UK: The Sydenham Society.

Tripathi, A. (2010). *The immortals of Meluha.* Chennai, IND: Westland Ltd.

Tubbs, R. S. (2019). "It is shameful for man to rest in ignorance of the structure of his own body" (Editorial). *Clinical Anatomy 32*: 861.

U

Upledger, J. E. (2009). *Craniosacral therapy study guide* (Rev. ed). Palm Beach Gardens, FL: The Upledger Institute. [Original work published 1987]

V

Varela, F. J., & Frenk, S. (1987). The organ of form: Towards a theory of biological shape. *Journal of Social and Biological Structures 10*(1): 73–83.

Vesalius, A. (1543). *De humani corporis fabrica libri septem.* Basel, CH: Ex officina Joannis Oporini.

W

Walsh, E. H. C. (1910). The Tibetan anatomical system. *The Journal of the Royal Asiatic Society of Great Britain.* October: 1215–1245.

Warwick, R., & Williams, P. L. (Eds.). (1973). *Gray's anatomy* (35th ed.). London, UK: Longman.

Y

Young, B., O'Dowd, G., & Woodford, P. (Eds.). (2014). *Wheater's functional histology* (6th ed.). Philadelphia, PA: Elsevier.

Acknowledgements

Whether they knew it or not, a great many people have, directly or indirectly, contributed to the making of this book. Even though there have been many more of you than can be individually named on this page, I am grateful and owe my thanks to you all.

My gratitude extends to include the myriad of sages and scholars who have, from times long past through to the present, had the clarity of vision to see the things they're looking at in a fresh light. Thank you for having the audacity to ask difficult questions, and then doing whatever it took to answer them in the ways that you did. For having the courage to speak publicly about your insights and discoveries, and for taking the time to record them in writing so they could be used by others in years to come. You are the giants upon whose metaphorical shoulders my work now stands.

The learning journey that led into the writing of this book has spanned quite a few decades. Along the way, my travels have been generously supported by a large number of talented teachers, lecturers, academic and clinical supervisors, peers and colleagues, technical and administrative support people, research participants, scholarship funders, peer reviewers, conference organisers, and publishers. Thank you for your help.

This quest would not have begun, however, nor have lasted this long without the help of two unassuming yet exceptional and very dear teachers – Keith Hubbard and Helen Nicholson. I couldn't have spotted the critical gaps in my knowledge and understanding, recognised the questions that needed to be asked, or developed the know-how and skills that led into the writing of this book without your perfectly timed guidance and support. Even though I wasn't always thrilled with your ability to spot my academic weaknesses and deficiencies, I am now profoundly grateful for every single bit of your gentle-yet-persistent nudging, stretching, encouragement, and testing. I thank you both from the bottom of my heart.

A deep and heartfelt set of thanks is also due to the many students, patients and clients who trusted my touch and my word, and from whom I learned so much. To the special few friends and family members who have resolutely stood beside me ever since you landed in my life, kindly tendering your acceptance and support, your love and encouragement have helped me to reach some of the crazy and seemingly 'impossible goals' I have set for myself … and have some tremendous fun along the way. Thank you, Jonny, for steadfastly holding on to your belief that this book (and the next one!) needed to and *would be* written someday.

As for the actual writing and production of this book, I would like to thank Dixie Carlton and Ann Wilson and the rest of their talented team at Indie Experts. My new friend and colleague Dixie is a 'word witch' and 'book midwife' extraordinaire whose Olympic brilliance, generosity of time, kindness, patience, and Kiwi-Australian funniness shepherded me through the transition from writing for an academic to a real-world audience (something that was much harder than it sounds). Ann, Dixie's behind-the-scenes book producing business partner, is pretty brilliant and funny too. Ann, masterfully abetted by the editing genius of Anne-Marie Tripp, did a great job of polishing the manuscript. I hadn't anticipated that the editing stage could be as easy and enjoyable (yes, *enjoyable*!) as it was. Daniela, for doing such a splendid professional job with creating the catchy book cover and other colourful artwork. Renée, for her artistry with the book design and layout. And Michelle, for getting me on-track with the 'book business' side of things. Thank you all, it has been a delight and privilege to have worked with you. Your pooled knowledge, enthusiasm, skills and hard work have helped make *The Living Wetsuit* what it is.

Thank you, Hilary Fogel, Bernie Landels, Rosie Ross, and Greg Cawley, for beta reading the first version of *The Living Wetsuit* manuscript. Your timely feedback about its readability and content was encouraging and helpful. Thank you, too, to the few brave souls who agreed to review the completed book and record their comments about it.

Last, but not least, to those of you who will take the time to sit down and read this book. I hope you will find it interesting and useful.

Te aroha,
Te whakapono,
Te rangimarie,
Tātau, tātau e.

The words of this Māori song (or *waiata*) are interpreted here as an acknowledgment and celebration of the love (*aroha*), the faith (*whakapono*) and the peace (*rangimarie*) that surround and connect us (*tātau*) … and make all things possible.

About Sue Adstrum

Sue Adstrum, PhD is an integrative anatomist (a transdisciplinary anatomy researcher and writer) who delights in demystifying anatomy so that people can be more constructively involved in the health-related decisions and activities that pertain to them, as well as the people they help care for. She graduated from the New Zealand School of Physiotherapy in 1974, and then, nearly two decades later, became fascinated by the relationship between anatomy, fascia (the body's soft connective tissue fabric), and the ways people *are able to* think about healing and healthcare. Wanting to learn more about these things, she enrolled at New Zealand's University of Otago as a 'mature' student and earned a string of useful postgraduate qualifications, ending with a PhD in 2015. Since then, Sue has written several widely-read journal articles, a textbook chapter, and has presented her research internationally at a number of conferences. Sue's work uniquely brings together several decades worth of conventional and complementary health practitioner training, clinical experience, and adult teaching experience with an eclectic raft of post-graduate university studies – in anatomy, anthropology, medical history and public health. *The Living Wetsuit*, her first book, pulls everything she has learned together in a way that she hopes will be accessible and useful for a general audience. To learn more about Sue, please visit: www.sueadstrum.com.